Narcissist

This Book Includes: Narcissistic Abuse & Dealing with a Narcissist. A complete guide to healing after emotional / psychological abuse, disarming the narcissist and understanding Narcissism

Dr.Theresa J. Covert

use or misuse of the information in question by the reader will render any resulting actions solely under their purview. There are no scenarios in which the publisher or the original author of this work can be in any fashion deemed liable for any hardship or damages that may befall them after undertaking information described herein.

Additionally, the information in the following pages is intended only for informational purposes and should thus be thought of as universal. As befitting its nature, it is presented without assurance regarding its prolonged validity or interim quality. Trademarks that are mentioned are done without written consent and can in no way be considered an endorsement from the trademark holder.

Table of Contents
Narcissistic Abuse

Table of Contents
Dealing with Narcissist

Narcissistic Abuse

Recovering from a toxic relationship and becoming the Narcissist's nightmare. Healing from emotional abuse and averting the narcissistic personality disorder to get your power back!

Dr.Theresa J. Covert

Introduction

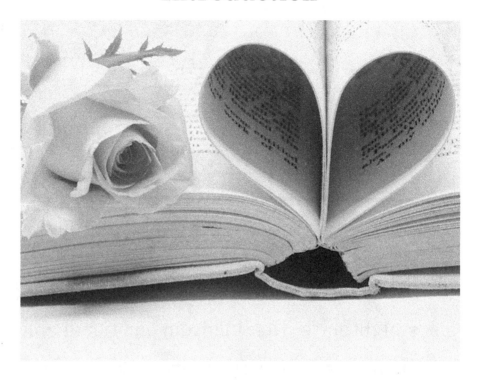

Congratulations on downloading *Narcissistic Abuse* and thank you for doing so.

The following chapters will discuss several topics related to identifying a narcissist, the signs of narcissistic abuse, the short and long-term effects of narcissistic abuse, as well as some tips for dealing with a narcissist and healing after abuse. There is really no way to describe how it feels to have dealt with a true narcissist; only those who have been affected and understand the depths of the abuse of a narcissistic will truly understand what it feels like. It is my hope that, through reading this book, that those who believe they've suffered at the hands of a narcissist or suspect the presence of a narcissistic abuser in their lives will be able to educate themselves so that they can identify and evade the chaos that awaits them.

In chapter 1, we will discuss the basics of narcissism and how the psychological community categorizes different manifestations of a narcissistic personality. We will then cover several different strategies and character traits which are trademark signs of a narcissistic abuser, including gaslighting and choosing targets. We will discuss what it is like to be in a romantic relationship with a narcissistic abuser and the effects of such abuse over time. Finally, we will look at some ways a person can protect themselves from potential narcissistic abuse as well as identify when they might be suffering from abuse and how to get help. The path to recovery from narcissistic abuse can be long and circuitous. The emotional and psychological effects often last for the rest of the person's life, but we must also remember that the human mind has an incredible capacity for healing and rebuilding.

There are plenty of books on this subject on the market, thanks again for choosing this one! Every effort was made to ensure it is full of as much useful information as possible, please enjoy!

Chapter 1: Understanding the Narcissist

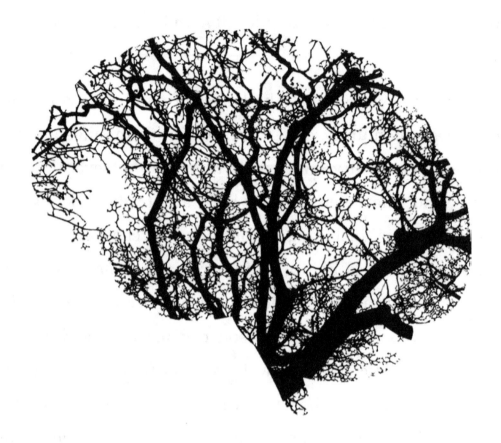

In order to discuss narcissistic abuse, we must first learn about the basic characteristics of a narcissist and how they manifest in their relationships with other people.

Many people will be surprised to learn that there are actually several different subtypes and manifestations of narcissism. For example, a narcissistic personality can be cerebral or somatic. The cerebral narcissist is the individual who believes they are intellectually much more capable and smarter than everyone else. They look down on others and assume as part of their nature that everything they have to offer intellectually is going to be much better than the others' contributions, whether it's an idea or plan of action at work or how best to do a job at home or in school.

The cerebral narcissist is all about impressing others with their mental prowess and may often exaggerate or even make up stories from their lives in order to inflate this reaction from other people. The underlining component to the narcissist's behavior, after all, is self-worship. They worship themselves, but they are also very needy when it comes to receiving praise from others as well. They will put others down if it makes them look better in everyone else's eyes without hesitation.

Then you have the somatic narcissist, who is basically just madly in love with their aesthetic qualities. They are generally very meticulous about their appearances and will do anything to maintain their looks. They are in love with their own reflections and see no faults when they look in the mirror. Think of the guy at the gym who seems to live there, constantly looking at his reflection and showing off for everyone around him. Whenever he sees someone else who looks good, he may go out of his way to demonstrate his superiority in some way. Now, this isn't enough to go on to concretely label someone a narcissist, but it would definitely be familiar territory in terms of how a somatic narcissist might spend his time.

When we talk about narcissism, I will most often refer to the narcissist as a "he." That's because it turns out, there are many more male narcissists than there are female. Psychologists have lots of theories and beliefs about why this is, and we can dig into that a bit deeper later, but know that in general, a narcissist is much more likely to be a man than a woman.

Okay, so we have these two overarching categories of narcissism. Now, let's talk a bit about the four different subtypes of narcissist personalities. These subtypes may be discussed using slightly different terminology in different mediums, but they are broadly uniform when we talk about the different types.

The first subtype is called overt narcissism. Overt narcissism describes a person who is narcissistic and openly displays this personality type. The overt narcissist is who most people think of first when anyone mentions the term narcissism. He is quite loud and boisterous about his personal accomplishments. She will use weapons like shaming and making fun of others in order to make herself look better than everyone else, especially when she feels like her status is being threatened. The overt narcissist does not hesitate to openly take action against others or to bolster their own egos without any regard to how it affects others. This is because one of the basic tenets of narcissism is a general lack of empathy for others. In their minds, there is no one more important than themselves, therefore, whatever they need to do to help themselves is perfectly fine, even if it means stomping all over others. This is often one of the first ways people recognize a narcissist; there is a blatant disregard for others that crosses over into inappropriate and hurtful territory, and they don't even try to hide it because there is zero feelings of shame or empathy. The overt narcissist will feed off of other people's positive reaction to their behavior, making them feel even more entitled to treat others how they want. They are the classic bully and may attract others as a kind of entourage simply because of the confidence and power they exude.

The second subtype of the narcissistic personality is called covert narcissism. This is an interesting one and probably quite controversial, depending on whom we're talking about. The covert narcissist is someone who hides their intentions and motivations behind a curtain of goodwill and humanitarianism. They contribute to charities, volunteer, help friends in need, but they do so with as much spotlight on them as they can conjure. They want to be seen being "good people" because this feeds their self-image of basically being a saint who can do no wrong. They relish the praise they receive from others, people telling them they are so nice and kind and generous when all they really care about is making themselves look good.

The third subtype and one of the most damaging to victims is the seductive narcissist. This applies to both romantic relationships and nonromantic relationships and refers to the emotional manipulation that takes place in order to tie a person to the narcissist individual through a toxic emotional addiction that is first cultivated through a showering of affection over time, and then suddenly withdrawn. The seductive narcissist is skilled at making his victim feel like they are the most important person in the world to him. He may give gifts and spend lots of money on dates and talk openly about his emotions, feign vulnerability and sincerity, then, once the victim feels attached, will suddenly withdraw, pulling his victim along behind him. This is an especially cruel situation because the victim is being used completely for the sole purpose of the narcissist's pleasure and self-worship. He may not have feelings at all for his victim, but simply enjoys having someone tethered to him under false pretenses. It is a sickening and deeply hurtful experience for the victim once they figure out what is going on if they ever do.

The final subtype is also one of the more damaging types and is the vindictive narcissist. Similar to the overt narcissist, the vindictive narcissist will be quite open with their narcissistic personality traits, but in addition, the vindictive narcissist is set on destroying and tearing down others. This is how they feed their need to rise above everyone else. Their victims could be family members, romantic partners, coworkers, or anyone else they come to view as "in their way" somehow. Their methods for tearing down and destroying other people include all types of emotional and psychological manipulation; whatever works best. They may plant insidious rumors about others in an effort to get people to hate one another or talk about people behind their backs in order to manipulate others' opinions of them. They are the playground bullies who love seeing those they deem weak cry and beg and get emotional. This makes them feel superior and justified in what they do.

In the next chapter, we will discuss how the narcissist interacts and affects those of us in the world we call "empaths." This is perhaps one of the most hurtful and toxic interactions that can happen in the world of narcissism because you are dealing with one individual who cares deeply and feels deeply in connection with others and one individual who is completely void of those feelings. When the narcissist gets his claws into an empath, the results can be devastating.

Chapter 2: The Toxic Attraction between an Empath and a Narcissist

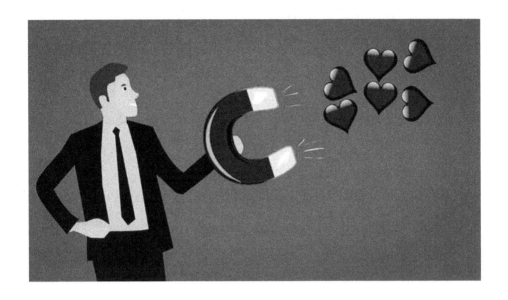

An empath is someone who feels not only their own emotions deeply, but the emotions of others. They are the people at work or at school that react instantly and intensely to both good and bad news shared by their friends and family. Some empaths use their empathic feelings to help others in their professional lives as therapists or in another medical field. Others, perhaps, feel a bit as though they are weighed down by their empathic feelings as they try to manage their own lives while shouldering others' emotions around them. We've all met someone who falls into the empathic category. It is one of the most wonderful experiences a person can have when he/she crosses paths with an empath and is able to form a friendship. This is because you always have someone you can talk to who is really going to understand and feel what you are going through, even if they haven't experienced the exact same circumstances. They understand and feel when you are sad, when you are happy, and everything in between. They are great fun to celebrate with because happiness is infectious and easily radiates into the empath.

There is a danger, though, especially when an empath is also prone to trusting her emotions more than her intellect or gut feelings. Empaths can be too trusting, especially if they are sucked in by someone who seems like they need support. This is where the toxic attraction between an empath and a narcissist can have dire consequences.

Let's demonstrate by painting a scenario. A young adult female is a demonstrable empath and is surrounded by a large group of friends as well as loving family members. She has never been purposefully hurt or manipulated because people love to be around her and value her as a friend. She's helped many of her friends through tough times in their lives through being there and providing a shoulder to cry on. She feels her friends' pain and is willing to go through it alongside them to help them through. When she sees someone in need, she feels very strongly for them and tries to help in any way she can. She is the girl you see going out of her way on the sidewalk to throw some change into the homeless man's bucket or help an elderly woman across the street or an elderly man with is groceries as he struggles to get them into his car. It is very difficult for her to simply ignore or do nothing when she feels someone else's pain or discomfort. Similarly, she is very sensitive to other people's feelings and expressions of anger and frustration. She avoids confrontation at all costs because the feelings are overwhelming for her. She often breaks down after a heated argument as she absorbs the feelings of anger given off by the other person.

Now, a narcissist happens to cross paths with this very kind, empathic person. It might be in a restaurant or at a bar when she is around her friends. He listens to bits and pieces of her conversations with others around her and picks up on the fact that she cares very deeply for the people around her, sharing in their pain and trying to help in any way she can. Perhaps, she sees her consoling a friend in a coffee shop while she almost seems more upset than the friend who actually went through the breakup, or some other situation. The narcissist ticks off items in a checklist which details his perfect victim. We can almost imagine him mentally checking off the boxes with a pen in his mind: naïve, gullible, kind, empathic, and trusting.

In this situation, different types of narcissists may adopt different strategies for making initial contact, and we will talk more about the process of how a narcissist chooses his targets in a later chapter, but for now, let's assume a narcissist decides to lure in this empath by subtly approaching and expressing some kind of sadness. He may hold his head in his hands, breath heavily, let out an exasperated sigh, any number of things to try and get this woman's attention. He may strike up a conversation and gradually work in that he is going through a tough time, gently suggesting that he wants to talk about his problems with her.

At this point, the narcissist is going to look for signals from the young woman. Is she comfortable around him? Does she feel intimidated? Scared? Is she still unsure and needs some more encouragement? Perhaps he picks up on some signals that she might be attracted to him. This is like getting a golden ticket for the narcissist and serves as his green light to work his way in further.

The narcissist, in this situation, is not going to be intimidated by her having friends around, either. One of the narcissist's overabundant character traits is overwhelming confidence in himself and his attraction. He's going to be able to tell when he's successfully intrigued this woman because it is all he cares about and looks for in other people. He is constantly trying out new strategies and gauging other people's reactions to his talk and behavior. At this point, even if her friends try to tug her away and bring the interaction to an end, the narcissist is going to sit tight and wait for the woman to come to *him*. He's already done his job.

Perhaps the woman, let's call her Claire, comes back a few minutes later to ask if he is ok or if he needs to talk more. The skilled narcissist might speak reassuringly to her while looking at her with eyes that suggest he appreciate having her around. He may make a subtle gesture, like touching her hand or arm, in order to gauge her new comfort level with him. He knows how to pretend like he needs support but does not want to interfere with Claire's fun night, which she will find endearing. The night will either end with Claire abandoning her friends in favor of helping out this attractive man who is clearly in pain and in need of support, or she will give him her number so that they may talk later. Either way, the narcissist can consider the play a win.

What is so dangerous in this situation is that the narcissist truly will feel absolutely no remorse for the emotional roller coaster he is about to put Claire through. He is going to revel in her attention and his ability to manipulate her emotions and actions toward whatever end he desires. He's going to know when he's managed to form an attachment that she feels is a real connection and when to pull back so that she craves being with him. He will work his way into her mind and perhaps even cause her to question her reality.

In the next chapter, we will discuss gaslighting—what it is and how it may be used by the narcissist. It is another effective tool which many narcissists learn to master because it offers so much in terms of being able to control another person's thought patterns and behaviors. You may have heard the term in relation to another form of mental manipulation called brainwashing. These terms refer to very real and very hurtful forms of manipulation that can lead to long-term confusion and emotional distress. We'll look at an example using the narcissist and our empath, Claire.

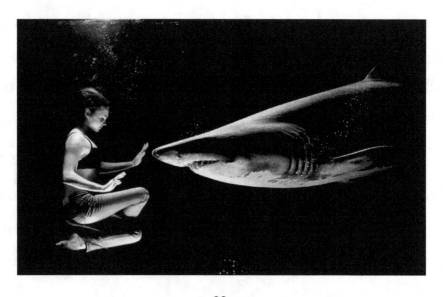

Chapter 3: The Gaslighting Narcissist

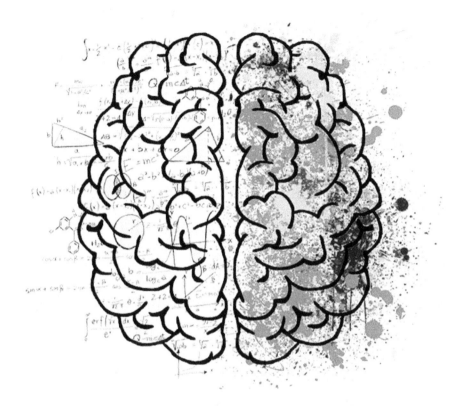

One of the things which make narcissism both fascinating and terrifying is that it can be difficult to work out exactly what makes them tick and what their specific motivations and objectives are. We know broadly that one of the main motivations for a narcissist in his life is to garner recognition and praise from others, but what about on a small scale, with an individual victim? Sometimes, it seems almost as though the narcissist is destroying a person's emotional health just for fun or to see how far he can go. It is a sick and depressing thing to think about. But what else could be motivating a person to treat another human being this way?

Perhaps, we can get a little bit closer by looking at some more of the fundamental characteristics of a narcissistic personality. We've already discussed the general lack of empathy, which pretty much applies across the board in terms of the different narcissist subtypes. But there is another important aspect of the narcissist which is the one thing he tries to hide more than anything, and that is insecurity.

It is important to note that people are not born narcissists, the personality is formed as a result of many different factors involving nature and nurture which are too complex and various to nail down on a general scale. However, when we look at a narcissist's history, it is sometimes possible to hypothesize as to what facets of his upbringing/childhood/adolescence may have contributed to his eventual turning into a narcissist. One of the reasons it feels so imperative to figure out why a narcissist is this way is the apparent meaninglessness and lack of reason involved in using emotionally manipulative tactics like gaslighting on another human being.

What exactly is gaslighting and how does it affect a victim over time?

Essentially, gaslighting is a manipulative process that, over time, causes the victim to question various aspects of his/her reality. To get a clearer picture of what I mean, let's look at some of the warning signs that someone is gaslighting you.

The biggest and most obvious telltale sign is when the person tells obvious, blatant lies. They may be able to look you straight in the face and tell a lie that you may or may not be absolutely sure is false. There is a calculated reason for the narcissist's confidence in himself and this tactic, and it has probably worked for him before. He is going to continue to lie to you until you start to question whether or not you actually know what's going on. People who are confident enough to lie like this, like narcissists, are going to be very effective in their delivery. It will be very difficult to counter their claims because they seem so sure about themselves and what they are claiming to be true.

Another warning sign occurs when the narcissists start to deny that they even said something when you know that they did. It's been said that if at any point in your relationship you feel the need to actually record a conversation, you should get your guard up because this is a pretty good sign that you're being gaslighted. The gaslighting narcissist will also use things and people that are precious to you and turn them into emotional weapons against you. They may back up their claims about you and your flaws with reasonable-sounding arguments, perhaps presenting them in a matter-of-fact way, as everyone knows about this except you. When they've managed to convince you that there is something wrong with you, just like they say, then they will continue to wear you down over time using other flaws or convincing you to isolate yourself from other family and/or friends, even your children.

It can be incredibly frustrating for the victim in a gaslighting situation because the perpetrator's words are often not going to line up with the person's actions. He will say things to you perhaps even lift you up and give you encouragement. But then his behavior may contradict what he has said to you, making you feel like his words are meaningless, or perhaps that you are doing something to cause him not to follow through with what he says.

Let's look at the example with Claire. Perhaps, after a few conversations, the narcissist, let's call him Mark, sees that Claire is growing more attracted to him. He has carefully constructed his story and conversation so as to portray exactly who he wants her to see, even though it isn't genuine. Let's say their relationship grows and he is able to convince her that there are some things about herself that she should work on. Maybe he brings up something about her personality that he overheard one of her friends' making a comment on. Mark begins to plant seeds of insecurity, doubt, and confusion based around the things that he knows she values. He may promise her the world, then seem to fall away completely until she comes begging for him to return to her. He then uses this opportunity of vulnerability to tell her that he would be a lot happier with her if she just fixed this or that thing, maybe it's her appearance or her job, or something else. Gaslighting comes into play when he begins to feed her lies and confuse her about the things that he has said which contradict his behavior. Any time she tries to call him out, he responds very confidently and convincingly, letting her know that she is incorrect. The key here is that he is going to make small steps toward this end over time. It is a slow burn, and Claire is going to suddenly find herself buried deep in her confusion before she even realizes what is going on. Things that she used to be so sure of will fall away and meld into the reality Mark wants to design for her.

The trap is insidious and can go on for years or even decades. The skilled narcissist knows that the more they can confuse you, the more control they can exert over you. They work to make you emotionally vulnerable so that you feel you need him to guide you through. Mark may take steps to turn even Claire's closest friends against her, and then blame them for all the emotional turmoil she is going through. At this point, Clair has developed an emotional dependency and feels like she is nothing without Mark.

The final straw, and the mark of success in the narcissist's mind would be to actually convince you that you are crazy, that you have no idea what you're talking about when you try to call him out on his lies or behavior. Once they can shut this down and make you totally question what's really going on around you, then they have complete control over you. They may feel like keeping up the charade and pulling you around further, or they may get bored and decide to move on to a completely new challenge, seeing as they've conquered you.

If and when Claire finally comes to the realization of what's been done to her, she may start to wonder, why her? What did she do to deserve this? For any victim of narcissistic abuse, this is a question that he/she will likely struggle with. After all, depending on how far the abuse has gone, the victim is going to have very low self-esteem and confidence, having been beaten down emotionally to feel worthless and stupid. So what is the answer to the burning question, why me?

Chapter 4: No Random Targets: He Chose You

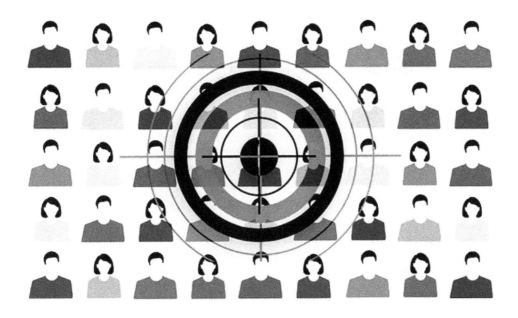

Make no mistake; the fact that a person is targeted has nothing to do with chance. In other words, the narcissist is not just going up to people randomly or based on one or two outward characteristics. The narcissist is a calculated thinker with a detailed plan in his head that is as natural to him as breathing. When a person is targeted by a narcissist, it is because this person fulfills many requirements which complete the picture of the perfect victim, similar to the checklist Mark was ticking off in his head as he observed Claire at the bar.

There are several characteristics and strengths which narcissists tend to target when they decide to break down another human being. Many people think that narcissists go after people who seem hurt or broken in some way. Well, this is both true and false. It's true that many narcissist abuse victims have some kind of pre-existing insecurity or source of pain in their lives, but this is not necessarily the main reason a narcissist would target them. You may think that because someone is weak, the narcissist is eager to make easy prey of them. But the truth is, most narcissists want to enjoy a challenge. Picking up an injured animal just to poke and prod an already broken-down creature would not be much fun or much of a challenge.

Instead, narcissists actually target those people who possess some aspect of personality or life circumstance that the narcissist doesn't believe they deserve or should have. It doesn't even have to be jealousy; a narcissist simply doesn't like seeing other people besides themselves find success or power. For this reason, the target of a narcissist may possess skills and character traits that define quite successful, strong people. The key is that their targets also ideally have a large amount of demonstrable empathy and compassion. In fact, the stronger and more intelligent the victim, the more satisfaction the narcissist is going to get from breaking them down.

So, let's complete the picture of an ideal narcissist victim. Of course, this isn't going to be a perfect example to fit every narcissist; there are going to be variances. But we know from research that the narcissist tends to target victims with certain sets of strengths and character traits.

Let's use Claire again as our example. We already know that Claire is an empath. She feels others' emotions as well as her own very strongly, and she feels that it is her duty to go out of her way to help others whenever she can. Let's say that she is also known to be someone with a lot of integrity.

Someone with high integrity is likely to be true to their word, hardworking, and honest with others. When they promise that they can make a deadline at work and it turns out to be a little tighter than they'd anticipated, they are going to work extra hard to make sure they follow through, even though they have to skip a meal or skip date night whatever they may have had planned before. This is an attractive trait for the narcissist because if he can successfully get his hooks in this victim, he knows he's going to be able to use feelings of obligation to coerce her into doing things she may not necessarily have done under different circumstances. Perhaps, he will be able to trick Claire into promising something based on an emotional need, then have to cancel other important plans that she's overlooked because she was preoccupied with the narcissist's incessant attention-seeking behaviors.

Claire, as an ideal victim, is also going to betray some source of emotional trauma or weakness which will make itself evident as the narcissist crawls his way into her mind. We can take a few pointers from the experiences of people who have fallen victim to cults.

One of the most effective strategies recruiters have used to get people too sucked into a radical new way of thinking in line with a cult is to find what it is that person is secretly desperate to find satisfaction for. Many people who are very lonely will latch on to a person and what they are saying simply in reaction to their showing the victim a measure of kindness and attention. There are many people out there who are so filled with pain and who feel isolated. When someone gives them an opportunity to find support for their pain, it is very easy for the person to also accept many other tenets and belief systems alongside that comfort.

Perhaps, a person who is down on their luck in the financial department comes upon a recruiter, whom he doesn't yet know is a recruiter, and this person starts a conversation. The recruiter commiserates with this individual, saying she also has some money issues. Then she goes on to say how she found relief through this group of people who work together and live together, relieving themselves of financial burdens connected with housing, transportation, etc. The recruiter makes it sound like heaven on earth, and soon, the man is brought in to the group and introduced to others. The source of the pain of the victim is always going to be addressed before introducing any kind of belief systems because it is imperative to hook the victim through emotional need before you can introduce new thought patterns.

The narcissist is going to employ a similar tactic in many instances, especially if they manage to get the victim to open up early in the interaction. There is nothing more thrilling to the narcissist than getting an otherwise strong, independent, and confident individual to open up about their vulnerabilities. The narcissist will use this information against the victim, playing up those things which tear the victim down emotionally, then building up a feeling of reliance and dependence on the narcissist to relieve these negative feelings.

If, after a few conversations with Claire, Mark has uncovered the fact that she's had a troubling childhood because of an abusive father, then Mark has a new set of shiny ammunition which is always available to tap in to whenever he needs to bring her down a notch or circumvent the defense mechanisms she has in place to deal with those old feelings. Mark will continue to gather and download information as he constantly observes Claire's behavior and mannerisms throughout their interactions.

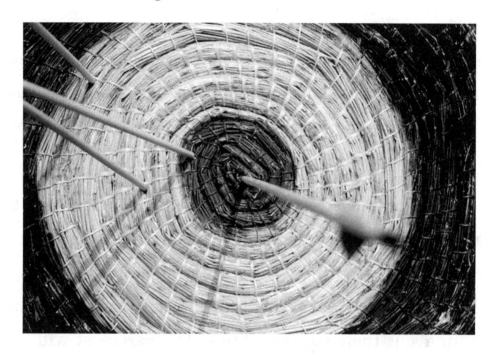

What's fascinating also is that the narcissist is going to be able to do his dirty work whether or not the victim is alone or with others. That's because he knows how to covertly exercise his strategies while in private so that they resonate even when they are with others whom the victim feels comfortable around. The narcissist may pull away from the victim in order to asses how long it will take for her to come back to him of her own free will, perhaps choosing to be with him instead of over with her group of friends.

This effect will grow gradually over time as he continues to cultivate a sense of dependency on his victims. Eventually, the victim will be so attached and confused that her other relationships may fall by the wayside.

So, we have an idea of the narcissist's modus operandi when it comes to one-on-one initial interactions, but how does the narcissist operate in general? What are some of the common mannerisms and behaviors that manifest in public or with family? In the next chapter, we will take a look at some of the ways narcissists behave and interact in various social settings.

Chapter 5: The Narcissist as a Social Creature

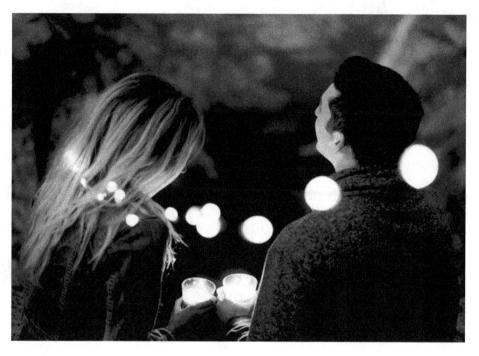

As we've established thus far, the narcissist is basically concerned solely with himself and his effect on others. It all seems like a game from the outside as onlookers analyzing the various behaviors and tactics narcissists employ. But for the narcissist, the reality is that she desperately needs the attention to cloak a likely very deep foundation of insecurity. This insecurity may stem from one of a thousand different experiences, but the root of the narcissist's drive tends to be a very deep need for constant admiration and validation, even though they don't value others in terms of intellectual capability. One can imagine the narcissist in the middle of a group at a party sharing knowledge on a given topic. Someone from the group compliments his thought process and the narcissist looks pleased for only a moment before scoffing audibly; he probably doesn't even know what I'm talking about, etc.

So what are some of the common social behaviors displayed by a narcissist? Let's look at several.

The narcissist is often knowledgeable, at least enough to impress himself and those in his immediate social circles. He may be loud and boisterous in an effort to show off his intellect, gaining favor from those around him because he seems like an affable, fun-loving guy. He will know how to work for a crowd and let them feel involved in the conversation only to captivate them with some pearl of wisdom or a carefully thought-through joke. The narcissist will want to maintain the façade of always being surrounded by friends who love being around him. His company may change often as he moves from one group to the next, entering and exiting conversations as he sees fit, always on the prowl for a potential victim who may be able to help him climb in some way. Underneath this façade is the fact that the narcissist is going to have very few if any, true friends. Aside from victims, the narcissist does not see friendship as necessary because he doesn't need anything from anyone. No one can offer him anything more than what he can offer himself over the long term. He refuses to interact with people who are mostly not as intelligent, and if he finds someone as intelligent, then he's going to do everything he can to destroy them or tear them down in some way. This is how he operates naturally. For whatever reason, he moves throughout the world on the constant lookout for ways to bolster himself above others while simultaneously tearing everything else around him down. Anyone who may initially try to cultivate a friendship will probably catch on to his superficiality quite quickly. The narcissist will only be able to fake intimacy for so long and to a certain extent because he truly does not feel anything for any other people.

In the work setting, the narcissist is going to know exactly who he needs to please and gain favor with in order to climb the corporate ladder. A skilled narcissist will know how to employ things like personality mirroring in order to make himself as amenable as possible to the boss or important coworker or supervisor. The narcissist is really going to know how to present himself in order to get themselves close to the people who are going to help them. But there are some triggers which are going instantly encourage a defensive or aggressive response, and these would be things to watch out for if you suspect someone to be a narcissist.

Oftentimes, a narcissist's stories or sharing of knowledge is going to be exaggerated or even made up in an effort to make himself look good. If the accuracy of this knowledge is challenged in any way, it's going to trigger a response of superiority and disdain, as if to say, what do you know about anything? Don't tell me I'm wrong, you have no idea what you're talking about, etc. Even if you confront the narcissist with point blank proof that their story is incorrect, they will defend themselves and insist that everyone else is lying or an idiot, etc. There is no end to the denial that a narcissist may employ to keep from ever admitting fault to any extent in nearly any situation. They never feel as though they owe anyone an explanation for their behavior. They will convey that they either believe you don't deserve to understand or you are too dumb to understand, etc. It is utterly pointless to try and argue a differing point of view with a narcissist because he is not going to respect you or care enough to try seeing things differently from his own point of view.

Within the family, there are all kinds of additional nuances and character traits which may stem from various earlier experiences in the narcissist's childhood. Let's look at an example.

Let's say that Mark was an only child and that he was pretty isolated throughout his childhood. His parents lavished him with gifts and gave him what he wanted in terms of money, but they never really spent much time appreciating who he was as a person or addressing him emotionally. Everything was about physical performance in sports of academic performance in school. He would get to go on expensive trips with groups from school and he would bring home trophies and the family would praise him and hang up his achievements all over the home, etc. But say he was struggling with a bully at school or felt sad about something someone said or felt insecure about some physical feature. His parents may have been dismissive and unwilling to address his emotional issues and let him wallow in his emotional pain without any support whatsoever. This could culminate, over time, in a sense that emotions don't matter, and since no one cared about how he felt, he has no desire to care about anyone else's feelings either. He may carry a sense of resentment toward his parents for the rest of his life, but because of the many praises he received for his academic and physical accomplishments, he also harbors a deep pride and sense of superiority over others. This is a great recipe for a future narcissist.

Oftentimes, the traits of a narcissist are overlooked by family members out of fear or simple denial. We know that it is quite common for parents to overlook the faults of their children, especially if they are a bit egotistical or even narcissistic themselves. If they are never at fault themselves, there is no way they could ever have a faulty child, after all. No, their children are quite perfect!

Overindulging a child in this way is also a good indicator of a future adult who is going to be overly arrogant and dismissive of others. The point at which arrogance crosses over into narcissism varies by person but always stems from foundational experiences, often consistent experiences over a long period of time, like overindulgent or under-indulgent parents. Only children are often subjected to feelings of loneliness, and if they are spoiled by the parents, they may gain a sense of entitlement that carries on into adulthood, coupled with a broken sense of empathy due to that prolonged isolation. Unfortunately, research has shown that in nearly 100% of narcissist cases, the narcissist will never be able to change and somehow learn how to "undo" the damage which led to their narcissism in the first place.

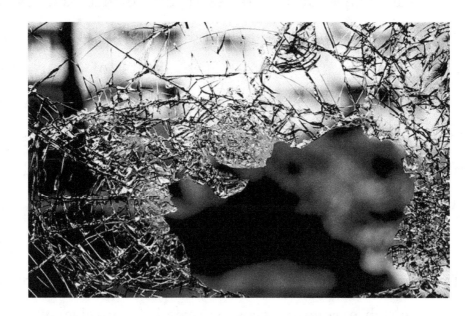

Chapter 6: Narcissism in the Relationship

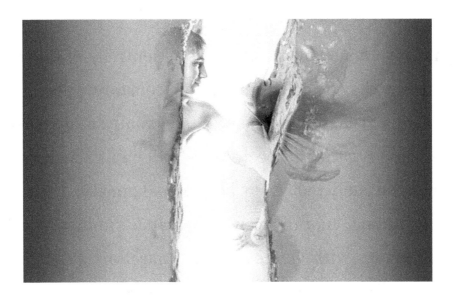

Now that we have a basic understanding of the characteristics of the narcissist and how he/she interacts socially on a broad scale, let's take a close look at how a relationship unfolds between a narcissist and an unsuspecting victim.

We will go back to our example involving Mark and Claire.

At the beginning of a romantic relationship with a narcissist, part of the scheme is that Mark is going to make Claire feel like she has found a regular Prince Charming. He will be everything for her and shower her with love and affection. He will give her everything she needs emotionally, and everything will seem perfect...for a while.

Remember what they say: If it seems too good to be true, it usually is.

This beginning "honeymoon" phase is essentially the hook that is designed to get Claire really craving his constant affection. He will give everything to her that she wants sexually and be everything she needs in every other respect. Mark will be like a drug, and soon she will become addicted, even before realizing it. Even the most upstanding, strong, morally conscious, and intelligent people are still human beings with desires. Skilled narcissists are going to get under your skin and learn your deepest desires in order to get their claws into you. Once this happens, you are at their mercy unless you pick up on the signs and run as fast as you can in the other direction!

But, unfortunately, Claire does not see any of the signs of narcissism because she has never met a narcissist who was trying to manipulate her. She never surrounded herself with people who were anything other than kind and compassionate, just like her. She loves that Mark has shown his vulnerable side, and he lets her feel like she is helping him through his pain, giving her a sense that she is giving as well as she is receiving. But over time, this will slowly fade away and reveal itself to not be the case any longer.

After a couple of months, perhaps, things will start to shift, as they always do. The timing will vary based on how the narcissist's plans are proceeding. But soon, the once overindulgent boyfriend is going to turn into something different, but at this point, Claire is madly in love with Mark, and what's worse, she trusts him. He starts to employ those emotional and psychological games which work to gradually tear down her self-esteem and confidence. He will introduce flaws and problems with her friends and family and incite arguments between Claire and the people in her life she loves and values. This will serve to slowly isolate her from those people she once trusted as she leans more and more on Mark, trusting in what he tells her because he otherwise gives her what she needs...until he doesn't.

The emotional games will gradually tear Claire down until she is just a shadow of her former self. The narcissist may have already employed gaslighting techniques or just now begin to introduce them as she focuses on the things that she now perceives are flaws in her character, her body, or her personality. Every now and then, she will get a glimpse of the Mark she knew when they'd first met, and this will keep her going for another period of time. But it will gradually start to dawn on her that things are not what they seem.

One of the first things victims in his situation might pick up on is the fact that the narcissist will be careless about consistency and repetitiveness because they do not care what others think or feel as a result. Mark will not necessarily value how his behavior in public reflects on Claire and may openly brag and show off and even flirt with other women right in front of her. When she goes to confront him about this behavior, he will easily deny it and tell her she is making things up—another symptom of gaslighting. It depends on the victim how far this will go. Some people are strung along for years and years. Eventually, the narcissist will simply disappear and then reappear sporadically, telling his victim that he is unsure about things and that he feels insecure about their relationship, perhaps pointing out things that the victim has done wrong in the relationship that makes him doubt her commitment, etc. The narcissist will use anything and everything at this point to inflict pain and make the victim feel like they need to make up for something they've done.

Eventually, the game is going to end, one way or another. Mark will have gotten bored with Claire and decided to move on. But oftentimes, the narcissist will not let go for a very long time, even if they are leaving for long periods of time in between their reappearances. Depending on how strong their chains have become connected to their victims, the victims will simply wait and hope and pray until the next time they see their narcissist partners. The emotional pain and control have run so deep that they do not feel they can live any other way.

When we think of women in physically abusive relationships, many people find it too easy to simply pass judgment on the women, suggesting that she just needs to leave, she just needs to leave... The fact is until you've experienced the kind of emotional abuse and manipulation exercised by an abusive partner, it is impossible to understand just how much a person can twist another human being's reality. Abuse victims often cite how they simply slipped into a state of denial or were so convinced that they were the problem in the relationship that they simply tolerated the abuse and blamed themselves for it happening. It is a sad but true reality. Don't ever pass judgment on an abuse victim until you really know what you're talking about. And even then, we must all realize that each one of us is very unique and that we all have different constitutions, strengths, and weaknesses. How many times have you heard it from someone that, they never thought they'd be dumb enough to fall for that, etc.

It's important to not internalize a feeling of being "dumb" if you've fallen victim to narcissistic abuse. The fact is that these people do nothing with their lives except getting better and better at manipulating and hurting others. They are professionals, and they are experts. You are not an idiot for being human and having feelings. You have simply run into someone who knows exactly how to take advantage of your common human decency and kindness.

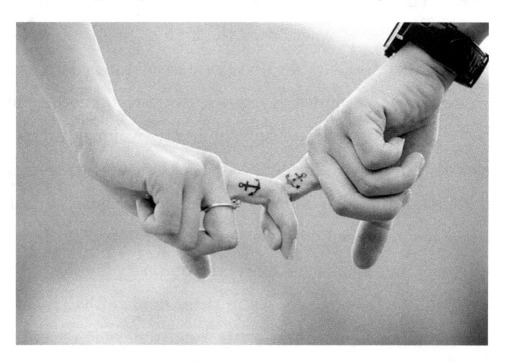

After the cycle of abuse ends and you've finally gotten free of the narcissist relationship, I hope that you can appreciate that you are lucky to have broken free at all. Many victims are strung along for the rest of their lives only to die in misery and in isolation without ever having received what they really needed and wanted from a romantic partner. What a victim goes through emotionally over the course of a narcissist abuse experience is harrowing and the effects are long-lasting. In the next chapter, we will talk about the emotional upheaval of ending a relationship with a narcissist and the effects of this experience in the long term.

Chapter 7: Effects of Narcissistic Abuse over Time

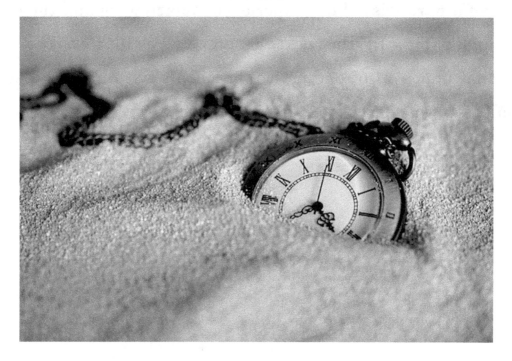

The effects of experience with narcissistic abuse can be devastating and long-lasting. Comorbid conditions like depression and anxiety are common after going through a period of emotional manipulation and may leave the victim with trust issues and anxieties that last the rest of their lives.

The signs of depression can vary from person to person, but the emotional turmoil caused by narcissistic abuse can trigger depression in people who have never experienced depression before in their lives. As a result of techniques like gaslighting, a person may begin to internalize a completely false reality about themselves, believing themselves to be flawed fundamentally, undeserving of love, and selfish. The narcissist understands that the more he can make a victim feel like they are doing something wrong, the more he can convince them to do things to correct the error or make up for what they've done. This is especially thrilling because the narcissist realizes that the victim has not actually done anything wrong; he's just that good at manipulation. It is really a matter of getting a notch on the belt for someone like the narcissist, and the effects on the victim do not garner any guilt or shame from him.

Depression manifests in a prolonged emotional state of hopelessness or helplessness. Many sufferers hear voices in their heads that constantly tell them they are worthless or stupid or that they are not enough. This voice may manifest as the narcissist's voice himself in a victim of narcissistic abuse. The voice may be persistent for days on end, especially at night when relaxation becomes impossible.

Anxiety is another possible aftereffect of narcissist abuse and especially common in instances where there is a history of physical abuse as well. The anxiety will often stem from the creation of doubt and destruction of self-esteem that goes along with narcissistic abuse. A once confident person may let down their guard just long enough for the narcissist to poke their head in and plant an idea about how that failed relationship was their fault, or they are really too fat to be wearing that, or that supervisor at work probably doesn't think you're good enough, etc. Whatever a narcissist can sink their teeth into, they will do it.

Towards the end of the abuse cycle, the victim may finally start to see the light and attempt to get as far away from the perpetrator as possible. This may or may not be successful, depending on what else the narcissist has going on at the time. He may have already found someone else to concentrate on, so you may find some peace and quiet, at least until they get bored and come find you again. Other times, the narcissist may completely disappear from your life without a trace and you may never hear from him again. This may initially feel tragic, as you've still got to deal with the emotional attachment that was cultivated. But soon, you will start to realize that you are a survivor of an abuser and you are lucky to be free.

One technique many abuse victims utilize after an experience like this is therapy, either in a group setting or a one-on-one setting. It can be very helpful to talk to others who have been through a similar situation and it is important to be able to ground yourself in the truth that you were not stupid or immoral or bad or not enough; you were manipulated, just like the others in your group. Talking to these individuals may go a long way in finding yourself again after a long and dreadful experience of narcissistic abuse.

There are several typical emotions and cycles of thought that victims of narcissistic abuse experience immediately following the end of the relationship. The victim is usually quite tired and worn out, and this may last weeks or even months. Emotional exertion takes a toll just like muscle exertion. It will take time to recover and heal from this stress. You may feel disgusted with yourself for having fallen victim to something like this. As I've stressed before, it is very important that you try to talk to someone or wrap your mind around the reality that you are not at fault. You are not stupid. Someone who is an expert at emotional manipulation with zero sense of remorse has taken complete advantage of you and your pain.

It is common for the victim to go through feelings of guilt and shame. Let these feelings run their course, but again, it is important to put yourself in an environment which supports the truth that you have survived an ordeal, not committed a horrendous crime.

Panic attacks and anxiety may go hand-in-hand for a while after the abuse. Some people get out without experiencing symptoms like this, but others will need to address the issue through talk therapy and/or drug therapy.

You will feel a big blow to your self-esteem, and this may take some time to build back up again. Try to surround yourself with people who love you and who care for you. You will likely go through all kinds of emotional fallout, and it is good to let it out when you need to. You may feel like crying or screaming or releasing your emotions in some other way. Perhaps, you may find it helpful to join a gym and go punch a punching bag for an hour. Whatever you need to do, try to express and release that emotion rather than bottling it up inside of you. This will only make the eventual release much worse and may even cause toxicity and additional emotional and psychological turmoil.

It will be natural to have a desire to think things through and figure him out. But it is important that you not exert too much effort on this, because the actions of a narcissist are contradictory, unreasonable, and sporadic. Narcissists do whatever they need to do to make themselves feel good at the time. If the next day they need to make a 180 and do something different, they aren't going to care whether or not it makes sense to you; they'll just do it. Don't try to figure them out. They're not worth it. And what's much more important; do not put yourself through the ordeal of thinking you can be an amazing enough influence that you can change them and make them not narcissistic anymore. I promise you, this is a waste of time. And likely they are going to use this as just another opportunity to manipulate you in some way. Believe me, cut your losses and move on. Don't ever look back. You may feel tempted from time to time to try and hunt this person down again. Maybe you want to tell them what they really did to you or try and explain to them what they've done wrong in an effort to gain some kind of affection or hint of the things they once showed you at the beginning of the relationship. It is so important that you realize that it was all an act—a complete façade. You must let these things go and move forward. And don't convince yourself that all men are awful and not worth the trouble. Relationships are always going to present unique difficulties, but I promise you that it is possible to find a partner who is respectful, loving, and who shares interests with you. Don't give up.

In the next chapter, we will discuss some tips for dealing with a narcissist in your life. Perhaps, this individual is a member of your family or someone who is simply not going away any time soon. There are ways you can compromise and deal with their existence in your life.

Chapter 8: Advice for Dealing with a Narcissist and the Aftermath of Abuse

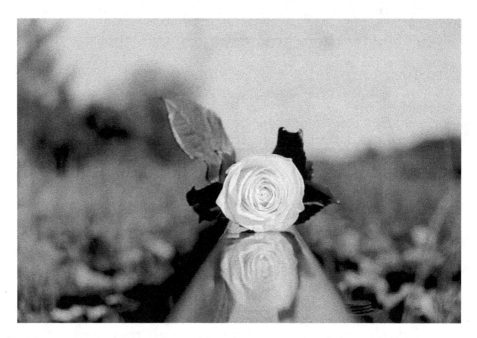

Before we address some advice for dealing with a narcissist and the aftermath of abuse, it is important that we outline some of the key indicators that you are indeed suffering from narcissistic abuse syndrome.

The first and foremost signal to yourself that you are suffering from dealing with a narcissist in a toxic relationship is the persistent feeling that you are alone. If you come home each day and see your boyfriend, eat meals with your boyfriend, sit in front of a TV with your boyfriend, then go to bed next to a boyfriend, but still feel like you've spent the whole day alone, it's because you might be dealing with a narcissist who is only presenting to you a mirage of the relationship you thought you were living. There is an absence of feeling underneath the actions that leave you feeling lost, confused, and very lonely. If you feel this constantly and are unsure of where the feeling came from, this may be a sign of narcissistic abuse syndrome.

If you are constantly struggling with the feeling that you are just not good enough for anyone, especially your boyfriend/partner, then you may be suffering from narcissistic abuse syndrome. Narcissists are very good at tearing down their victims' self-esteem and convincing them through both subtle and not-so-subtle strategies that they are messing things up, constantly making mistakes, etc. They may make fun of you and laugh at you or mock you and make you feel small. This abuse leads you to believe that you are worthless and that you would never be good enough for anything you want to accomplish in life.

You may feel suffocated by the relationship itself as your narcissist partner attempts to hijack your personal life and everything that existed before he/she entered your life. It is a trademark strategy of exercising control to isolate the victim from those he/she once trusted and loved. It is the narcissist's goal to make him/herself the only person you lean on for anything kind of support.

Another sign of narcissistic abuse syndrome is the realization that you've become a different person in terms of belief systems, morals, principles, or other characteristics which were once at the core of who you are. If your partner has managed to change these essential things about you and they don't seem right, it is a sign that you've got some toxic forces at work doing everything they can to make you into a different person that serves the purposes of only the narcissist.

Narcissists often utilize outright name-calling in an effort to belittle and gradually break down a victim's sense of self-worth. This practice may not be overt in the beginning, but instead, be framed as a kind of joke and kidding by the narcissist. He may say while giggling, "You're just overreacting because you're too sensitive." Comments like these may seem innocent at first, but over time with persistent use, these things can be internalized by the victim until the accusations became a reality for them. They may start to believe these things which at first they didn't feel were affecting them in any damaging way.

Finally, the cycle of something called "hurt and rescue" can take such a toll on a victim as to lead to life-long emotional anxieties and struggles. With this technique, the narcissist introduces stress through an event or an argument or an accusation and then gives the victim the silent treatment for a certain amount of time. They may use a tactic other than the silent treatment, but whatever they choose to do, the object is to relieve that stress or silence it for an amount of time. The silent treatment, when used in this way, triggers a fear of abandonment that is innate in pretty much every human being out there. This makes it an inescapable strategy to induce pain, as long as the victim feels attachment and emotion for the perpetrator.

The rescue stage entails the perpetrator coming back and relieving that fear of abandonment, but now, the victim has learned to be afraid whenever the cycle starts again, anticipating that period of staged abandonment, or silence.

Over time, this technique becomes a powerful strategy for control and manipulating behaviors because the feelings associated with abandonment can be so strong and hurtful. Each one of us is hardwired to crave attention, love, and affection, so when someone offers this then abruptly takes it away, we learn to do whatever we need to do to avoid having that attachment leave us again, even if it means apologizing for something we didn't even do, much to the narcissist's delight.

When you feel sure you are dealing with a narcissist in a romantic relationship, you need to seek support in getting out and away as soon as possible. Educate yourself on the tactics used by narcissists to keep that feeling of attachment in you and do everything you can to resist it and break free. Remind yourself again and again that it's all been an act and nothing you were feeling attached to is real.

If you are dealing with a narcissist who is not a romantic partner but still an unavoidable part of your life, your best defense is going to be constant awareness and alertness to any schemes and manipulation the narcissist may be trying to employ on you. It would be unwise to start an all-out war on the narcissist since his whole being is centered on crushing others and he will surely be able to invest more time and emotional energy into hurting you than you will in hurting him. Besides, you're not that kind of person!

Even though you may feel anger, letting your guard down and losing control is exactly what the narcissist wants you to do, so do not give him the satisfaction.

As always, strength in numbers is a good rule of thumb to follow. If you are feeling vulnerable or susceptible to a narcissist in your purview, recruit others to support you and help form a barrier. Let the narcissist know that you are too smart to fall for his schemes and that you are not going to give an inch. Create a thick skin around yourself and prepare for some demeaning insults designed to rile you up. You don't have to give in to these. Form your support group and move on with your life. When the narcissist sees that you've all but become immune to his charms, he will look elsewhere and leave you alone. Be on the lookout for others whom he may be targeting and be sure to let them know what's going on if you think they are also in danger. This will probably trigger a defensive response, but the key is to maintain your composure and remind yourself of your reality and your standing. Don't buy into the narcissist portraying himself as more than what he is. Inside, he is just an insecure little boy trying to validate himself through other people's praises. He does not have power over you or those you love. You are stronger than this person because you know the strength and power of genuine love and affection.

In our final chapter, we will discuss some advice and tips for those who have gone through the abuse from a narcissist and are on the journey towards recovery. We will also discuss how you can arm yourself against future narcissist abuse. As always, I encourage you to educate yourself as much as possible about the narcissist and his various schemes. Knowledge, after all, is power.

Chapter 9: Recovery

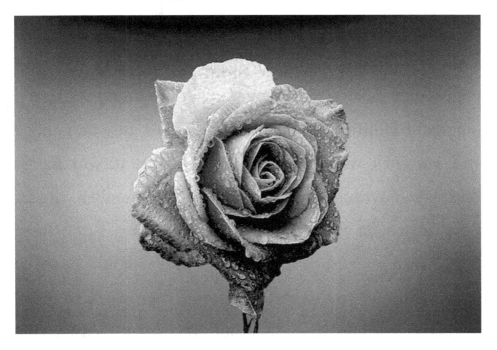

I believe strongly in the power of self-healing, and I believe that any degree of emotional pain can be addressed through self-care and healing practices over time. It may be a long road and will certainly not be easy, but with proper support and belief in yourself, it is possible to move past the experience of narcissistic abuse to a large degree. You may not be able to erase the effects entirely, but it is possible to move and live a healthy, productive, and emotionally stable life after even the most damaging of emotional experiences. This is because the human brain has an incredible capacity to rewire itself and relearn how to live and love through healthy habits and new thought cycles that will take the place of the old, destructive thought cycles.

First of all, grab an old journal or buy yourself a nice new one. Many survivors of abuse can attest to the power of simply writing out and processing your feelings through words. There may be many aspects of your experience with narcissistic abuse that you have yet to really address or wrap your mind around. Remember, the key here is not to focus on figuring out or working out the mental manipulations of your abuser. The focus here should be on working through the feelings you experienced and then work to disentangle those negative feelings from the thought cycles feeding them. For example, you may have heard your abuser constantly accusing you of being too fat or too skinny. Write about how this made you feel, then reinforce the fact that there is nothing wrong with your body and that this was just one of many tools your abuser used to break you down. Letting these feelings bring you pain over and over is simply a type of surrender to your abuser. Replace these negative thoughts with positive, affirming thoughts about your beautiful body and what it has done for you. Expressions of gratitude can also go a long way to dispel feelings of worthlessness and emptiness. Again, it won't dispel all of your negative feelings right away. Forming positive habits of thoughts takes time, but it is well worth it. Don't let the incessant negativity from your past relationship dominate your future thoughts.

Another way to help you process and move through negative emotion to release this energy is through physical exercise or contemplative movement therapy, like yoga. There are many yoga practices designed specifically to help you move your thoughts through negative emotions into a more positive space. Cultivating a healthy body leads naturally to encouraging a healthy mind and thought habits.

Don't be afraid to lean on support sources. It is going to be very important, especially in the first few weeks or months following a traumatic emotional experience, to be able to lean on others for support. Perhaps, your experience with narcissist abuse has left you alienated from friends and/or family. Now is the time to reconnect with those loved ones. Don't be afraid. They are probably going to be so excited to have you back they won't even press you for details. Simply accept their support and love and lean on it when you need to. When you are ready, ask if you can discuss some of the details of your abuse as a way to process and move through them.

Educating yourself about narcissists and their tactics is going to be very important as you want to arm yourself against future abusers.

If you feel you were too quick to trust in your last relationship, you may need to practice setting up barriers and waiting for people to prove to you that they are trustworthy. This may be difficult for those people who are naturally generous and giving of themselves emotionally. This can be a wonderful and amazing trait, but it is important to realize that not everyone you meet is going to have good intentions. Hopefully, you never have to meet another narcissist again. But if one should cross your path, it won't hurt to have educated yourself about how exactly to spot one and move away from that influence.

One of the most important things you can do on your path to recovery to ensure your success is to forgive yourself and let go of those feelings of guilt and shame. It won't be easy to simply dismiss these feelings, especially if you've spent months or years listening to someone tell you you're not good enough or not smart or flawed in some way. This is going to take time to move away from, but it is important to make a daily habit of verbally or internally reaffirming that you are a survivor of narcissistic abuse and that you were strong enough to pull away.

Meditation can be a very helpful tool throughout this process. Begin by sitting comfortably in a space that is quiet and free of distraction.

Practice breathing slowly and taking deep breaths each time you breathe in. Focus on your body in space and feel each part of your body as you breathe. There are several guided meditations available online for you to peruse if you so desire, or you may choose to come up with your own little mantra. Whatever you decide to do, try to make some time each and every day to focus in on your affirmation. Repeat the words to yourself slowly, over and over. Tell yourself that you love yourself, that you forgive yourself, that you are enough, that you are loved, that you are strong. Simply saying these words to yourself will begin to break the toxic habit and thought cycles that once plagued your mind and triggered anxiety. Eventually, you will come to a place where those negative feelings are no longer connected to the obsessive thoughts that intruded on your mind. As you practice replacing these bad thoughts with positive ones, it will become habitual and begin to feel more natural. Meditation can be kind of strange for first-time practitioners, but I encourage you to give it a try if you are struggling to move past those negative obsessive thought cycles.

Finally, do what you can to cultivate a regular sleep schedule where you get at least 8 hours of sleep. Setting aside some time at night before bedtime for meditation may be a great way to help your brain settle down and prepare for rest. Try to go to bed at the same time every night and do something calming right before. Try not to eat and snack on junk food late at night as this will keep you up longer and may disrupt your sleep.

Know that you are strong enough to move past this horrific ordeal and that you are not alone in your experience. Re-learn to love and take care of yourself and reaffirm each day that you are worth the effort of recovery.

Steel yourself should your abuser ever re-enter your life for any reason. Enforce strict boundaries and enforce a rule of no contact whatsoever. Do not answer phone calls, texts, anything. He is not worth it, and there is nothing positive that he can offer you. You have risen above that influence.

Conclusion

Thank you for making it through to the end of *Narcissistic Abuse.* Let's hope it was informative and able to provide you with all of the tools you need to achieve your goals whatever they may be.

The next step is to share what you have learned with anyone else in your life or your family's and friends' lives who you think may benefit from the information on narcissistic abuse offered in this book. As I've said many times throughout this text, the most important weapon you have against narcissistic abusers is knowledge and learning how to spot them before they have a chance to harm you. If you or someone you love has experienced narcissistic abuse firsthand, I hope that the information and advice in this book have offered some degree of comfort and help as you move forward past this awful experience. People suffer each and every day at the hands of narcissistic abusers, and it is more important now than ever before that we all help spread the knowledge and tools available to defend ourselves from potential abusers. It is possible to escape, even if you've already fallen victim. Don't underestimate the power of the human mind to overcome even the most hurtful of emotional experiences. As you wake up each morning and take steps toward recovery each day, I hope you remember the encouragement and the tips offered in this book. Also, don't be afraid to get creative and realize new ways that are personally helpful that you may be able to share with others who may share in your unique experience. There are many different ways survivors can choose from on their paths to recovery. The key is to believe in yourself and trust in your instincts and gut feelings fueling you forward and past any and all symptoms of narcissistic abuse.

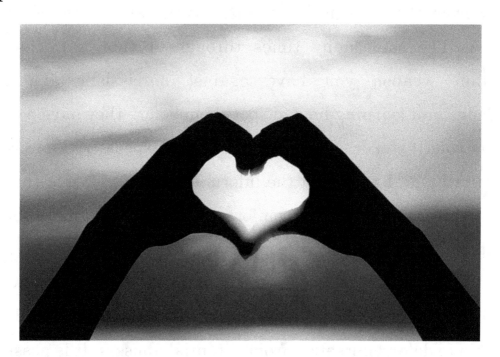

Dealing with a Narcissist

Disarming and becoming the narcissist's nightmare.

Understanding Narcissism & Narcissistic personality disorder.

Healing after hidden psychological and emotional abuse

By Dr.Theresa J. Covert

Introduction to Narcissism

The following chapters will discuss various tips and tricks that can help you deal with narcissistic people in your personal life and your career, but before we go into that, let's briefly introduce the concept of narcissism.

The term "narcissist' can be used to describe a fairly wide range of people. Narcissism could be manifested in a mild form in a leader who is charming and charismatic, but also a bit egotistical. On the other end of the spectrum, it could be manifested in a person with a "narcissistic personality disorder." Such a person would be grandiose to the extent that he/she gets violently angry if you don't give him/her attention or admiration.

The fact is that narcissism exists on a spectrum and even the nicest people tend to have mild narcissistic tendencies. For this book, we will be discussing how to deal with the sort of people in whom narcissism is manifested as a major personality trait.

We mistakenly attach the "narcissist" label on people who have high self-esteem, or people who talk with great pride about their careers or their personal lives. Such people aren't necessarily narcissists in the clinical sense of the word.

Narcissistic people are those who feel that they are special (more than anyone else around them), that they deserve a lot of appreciation just for giving us the time of day, but most significantly, they have a diminished sense of empathy towards others. Narcissists also have lots of other negative attributes that branch out from these main ones, and those attributes make them incapable of fulfilling other people's needs in relationships.

Narcissists aren't oblivious of the fact that they are self-centered. They are consciously aware of their selfishness, but they truly believe that the selfishness is warranted because after all, they think they are special.

Narcissists expect people to give them special treatment, so they actively manipulate and control people to ensure that they satisfy that need. Therein lays the problem for most people. If you have narcissists in your life, you can rest assured that they will try to get you to give them special treatment, because they just can't help it.

If you want to avoid ending up under the thumb of a narcissist, then reading this book is a great first step for you.

There are plenty of books on this subject on the market, thanks again for choosing this one! Every effort was made to ensure it is full of as much useful information as possible; please enjoy!

Chapter 1: Understanding the Mind of a Narcissist

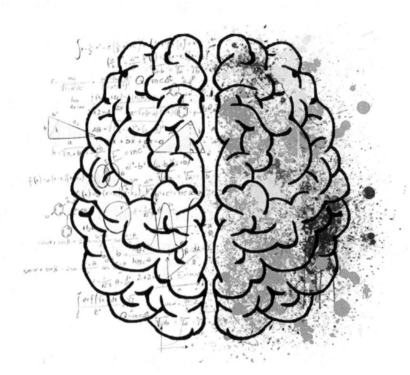

There is a common misconception that narcissists are people who love themselves a lot. In actual sense, they are people who love the way other people perceive them, and some of them actually dislike or even loathe themselves. The terms 'narcissism' and 'narcissist' come from the name 'Narcissus.' Narcissus is a character in Greek Mythology. He was a handsome hunter who was cursed by the gods to live without human love, and in the end, he could only fall in love with a reflection of himself. Like the original Narcissus, people with narcissistic personality traits don't fall in love with other people, but they instead fall in love with versions of themselves that you mirror back to them.

Narcissists are known for self-flattery. They often brag about everything, and they are insistent on making themselves seem superior to everyone else around them. That doesn't necessarily mean that they love who they are, or that they are striving for perfection in order to better themselves. More often than not, the vocal self-assuredness and the arrogance is usually a cover for a deep self-hatred that they aren't willing to open up about.

Some narcissists aren't even willing to admit their self-loathing to themselves, so they live under the delusion that they are better than everyone else and that they are immune to the shortcomings that everyone else suffers from, or that they are above almost everything. To most of them, arrogance is, in fact, a way to cope with their own shortcomings.

Narcissists tend to treat others with a lot of disdain, but that disdain is meant to conceal jealousy. If someone else is the center of attention, you can be sure that the narcissist will try to one-up him/her, and if that is not possible, the narcissist will try to criticize the person or diminish the accomplishment in one way or the other.

Narcissists often look outwards in their criticism of others, but they are very afraid to look inward to examine their own talents and attributes. Deep within, narcissists know that the truth about their own condition is quite devastating. They will make claims about how good they are at something, or how better they are than other people, but they will do everything necessary to prevent you from examining their claims too closely.

From an emotional standpoint, narcissists are dead inside. There is an emotional emptiness in them, and they are often looking to fill that emptiness with external validation. If you are around a narcissist or you are in a relationship with one, all they are going to do is seek constant validation from you. When they lie to make they seem smarter or more accomplished, it's in service of seeking respect and validation from you. If they keep trying to manipulate you emotionally, it's because they want to control the way you perceive them for the purposes of validation. If they react angrily or violently in certain situations, it's because they feel like they are not getting the validation they were hoping to get from you at that point in time.

The irony is that although narcissists are always looking for validation, they can never give it to other people. You know that

human relationships are based on reciprocity, so
validation to someone, they are more likely to give it ba.
Narcissists want you to validate them, but they will never
you (unless they are trying to manipulate you). Narcissist. are
incapable of appreciating love, so if you express love (or any other
positive emotion) towards them, they will either alienate you or they
will trample all over that love.

To fully understand the narcissistic mind, let's look at the
diagnostic criteria that are used by mental health professionals and
psychologists to identify them. Here are the nine main
characteristics of narcissists:

1. They feel a high level of self-importance, and they often
   exaggerate their capabilities and their accomplishments.

2. They dream of having unlimited control, power,
   attractiveness, intelligence, and success.

3. They think they are special and one-of-a-kind and they want
   to be associated with high-class people or entities.

4. They are always looking to be excessively admired.

5. They are always looking for special treatment, and they
   always expect you to comply with their wishes or demands.

6. They won't hesitate to take advantage of your for their own personal gains.

7. They don't empathize with others. It's always about them, so they won't go out of their way to accommodate your needs.

8. They are always jealous of others, and they wrongly believe that others are jealous of them.

9. They are very arrogant, in both their words and their actions.

Now, we all may have one or more of these traits in us, but narcissists are those who tend to have most of these traits and to exhibit them constantly.

Chapter 2: Identify the Type of Narcissist You Are Dealing With

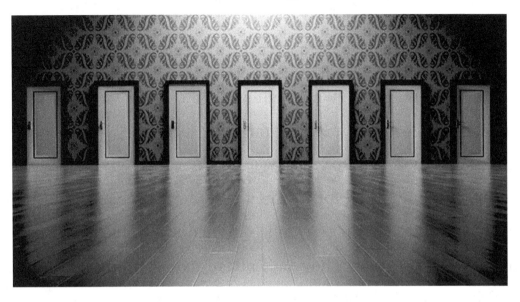

Narcissism manifests itself in many different ways, so there are many types of narcissists. You can categorize narcissists according to the way they act in relationships, or according to the traits that they manifest more often. In this chapter, we will look at the five main types of narcissists. If you spend a lot of time with a narcissistic person, you may find that they show signs that fall under more than one of the categories we will discuss in this chapter, but when you want to figure out which category a particular narcissist falls under, always go with the one that covers his/her most dominant traits. Here are the five main types of narcissists that you are likely to deal with at some point in your life:

The Know-It-Alls

These are narcissists who believe that they are always the "smartest guy in the room," and they are very concerned with making sure that everyone knows it. They will give their opinion even when no one asked for it. They will insist on being the center of the conversation, even if the topic under discussion is clearly not in their area of expertise. They will often give you advice that seems helpful in their minds but is of no actual value to you.

These narcissists also make for terrible listeners because, when it's your turn to speak during the conversation, instead of paying attention to what you are saying, they are always thinking about what to say next. They are always ready and willing to offer you long lectures, just to let you know how much they know, and they have a difficult time letting anyone else speak.

The Grandiose Narcissists

These are the kind of narcissists that always wants to appear more important and more influential than anyone else. They never shut up about their accomplishments, and they are always trying to convince people that they are more successful than they actually are. They are always looking to gain the envy and the admiration of others.

These narcissists always believe that they are destined for greater things than anyone else around, and they may act in a selfish way because they believe their special status entitles them to preferential treatment. In fact, they think that if they receive preferential treatment, it is in service of some kind of social good. They believe that they belong at the top of the pyramid of some sort of social hierarchy, whether it's at work, or at home.

One interesting thing about grandiose narcissists is that sometimes, their grandiosity can be a self-fulfilling prophecy. Some of them are more driven, and also a bit charismatic as a result of their grandiosity. In the end, that causes them to succeed. Sometimes, people may start to revere them, and they may put them in positions of power.

The Seducers

These are narcissists who tend to manipulate people for their own benefit. Unlike other narcissists, these ones may actually make you feel good about yourself, but that feeling never actually lasts — it ends as soon as they get what they want.

Seducers will start off by expressing admiration for you, but it's always just something that they think you want to hear, and the point is to get you to offer them the same admiration so that they can take advantage of you.

Once the seducers have gotten what they want from you, they reveal their true colors, and they pull the rug from under your feet. Such a person may keep offering you compliments, but the moment you comply with their request, they start giving you the cold shoulder.

If you are dealing with a person who keeps flattering you, try to see if he/she does the same with everyone else. If the niceness is only directed towards you, the reason could be that they are targeting you for manipulation.

The Bullies

These narcissists work under the assumption that one builds himself or herself up by tearing down or humiliating others. The purpose of bullying is to assert one's superiority, and this kind of narcissist is really brutal in the way he/she does this. We are not talking here about the school-yard bully – the narcissistic bully is a lot more sophisticated than that (although his/her methods may be somewhat similar to the ones of the school-yard bully).

This kind of narcissist treats others with contempt, in the hope that they will feel like losers, allowing him/her to feel like a winner in the process. This is the kind of person that will disparage you at every turn, and he will undermine and pour cold water on all your efforts at self-improvement. Their criticism is never constructive — it is meant to mock you and tell you that you are not capable or worthy of improvement. When this type of narcissist wants something from you, he/she doesn't ask for it, he/she demands it; as though it's something you owe him/her.

The Vindictive Narcissist

This is the kind of narcissist that is out to destroy you. This narcissist is destructive by nature, and to him/her, everything and everyone that challenges their superiority have to be brought down.

These narcissists tend to target people for reasons that the average person would consider mundane. They hold grudges that are completely one-sided. These are the kinds of people who think of you as their ultimate nemesis just because you stepped on their toes by accident a few months ago.

The vindictive narcissist can't let anything go, no matter whom silly it may seem to you. If it's someone in your social circle, he/she could trash-talk you to your friends or family (in your absence) just to make you look bad. If it's a colleague, they may make up stuff about you in an attempt to get you fired. If it's a former spouse, he/she can try to turn your kids against you. They may pose as victims to make you look like some sort of predator, or to make you look "crazy."

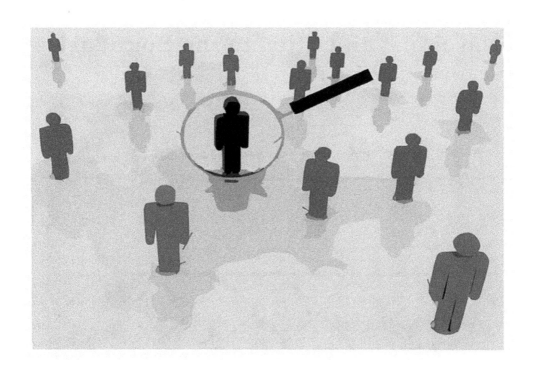

Chapter 3: Create Boundaries with the Narcissist and Stick to the Boundaries

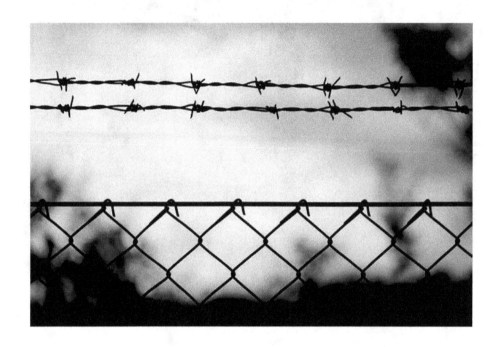

You have to know where to draw the line with the narcissistic person. You have to decide beforehand what sort of behavior you are willing to put up with, but you also need to have strict rules for yourself about the things that you aren't willing to tolerate. Don't just go in with vague mental boundaries. In fact, wherever you can, you should create clear, well-defined boundaries, write them down, and do everything in your power to enforce them. Unless you have clear boundaries, a narcissist will walk all over you, and you will be stuck making excuses for his/her behavior.

One area where we have difficulty setting boundaries with narcissists is in the amount of time and attention that we give to them. In our minds, we always feel the need to stick around and keep interacting with anyone who tries to talk to us. It's like they have this strange ability to hold us hostage. That means that you have to make a conscious effort to resist the urge to be complacent when a narcissist hogs your time. If for instance a narcissist keeps talking on the phone when you have important things to do, just say you have to go and hang up before he has the opportunity to talk you out of it. As we've mentioned, they demand a lot of attention, and unless you set limits, they won't stop.

When you set a boundary with a narcissist, you can rest assured that they are going to test that boundary, and they are going to push it as far as you will let them. So, you have to go in with the conviction that your boundaries are not up for discussion. For example, the narcissist who keeps hogging up your time will try out all kinds of tricks to keep you talking to them, to see if you are flexible on the boundary that you have set.

For the narcissist, it's all about control, so he/she will do everything imaginable to regain control over you once you've set the boundary. He may try to convince you that you are unfair to him by denying him attention. He may try to argue with you, intimidate you, guilt you, or even confuse you. If you show any kind of flexibility, he will keep pushing at it until he knocks down your boundary. It may seem rude on your part, but if the narcissist insists on talking to you on the phone when you have made it clear that you don't have the time, just say bye and hang up.

When you set your boundary, don't explain yourself more than once. Let's take the example of a narcissist that keeps insulting you during an interaction. In this case, you will set a boundary by telling him that if he keeps being disrespectful, you are going to walk away. Of course, he is going to test you by insulting you again. Once he does this, put your money where your mouth is and walk away.

If you explain yourself a second time, that is a concession, and it will have a domino effect, and the end result will be detrimental to your stance. A narcissist will violate your boundaries intentionally, and he will always have a ready excuse to explain why that violation was warranted. If you tell him not to call you late at night, he will call, and he will pretend that he totally forget about your warning. So, when the phone rings despite your warning, ignore it. If someone pretends not to remember something you explicitly asked them not to do, they are manipulating you.

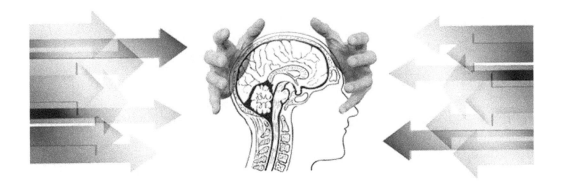

You have to remember that you don't have to explain yourself or to justify your actions to anyone. They are not the boss of you, and they don't get to interrogate you on matters that are personal to you. If you feel like saying "No" to someone over anything, it's entirely up to you to decide if you want to explain it to them (unless it's your boss at work, and even then, there are limitations to that). You have to understand that any information you offer to a narcissist will be used against you in that interaction (or in future interactions).

Narcissists always believe that they are more important than you, so to them, your boundaries are always up for review. So, you have to remember that setting and enforcing boundaries with narcissists isn't a one-time event. If it's someone that is in your life, you have to stay vigilant and to enforce your boundaries consistently. For example, if you ask a narcissist to stop hogging your time, he may stop temporarily, but a few days later, he will start testing the waters to see if you have loosened your stance. When you set your boundaries, be mentally prepared to deal with the fact that the narcissist will keep trying to abolish them for as long as you keep associating with him/her.

Chapter 4: Empathic Validation

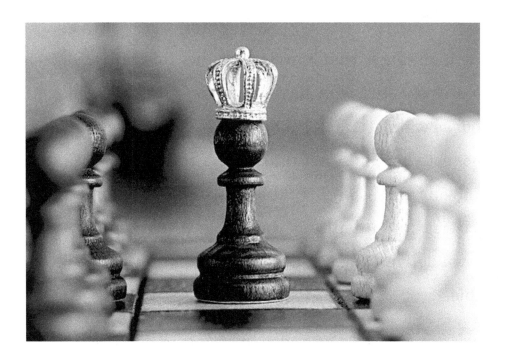

When dealing with a narcissist, you have to be very careful about how you criticize his/her behavior or actions. Narcissists don't deal well with criticism. Although they are great at dishing it out, they are extremely thin-skinned when they are the ones being criticized, and they may lash out in ways that could harm you a lot more. So, to be able to criticize a narcissist effectively, you should learn to use emphatic validation.

Emphatic validation is a technique used to deliver criticism by concealing it in the midst of compliments. Most people are receptive of critical notions about them if the criticism is sandwiched between 2 compliments.

We have mentioned that narcissists live for validation, so if you want to criticize one, you have to make sure that the criticism is disguised as validation. It's not that we don't want you to value brutal honesty here; it's just that we are trying to get you to be more tactful in your approach. Brutal honesty will only serve to aggravate the narcissist, and it will put you in his/her crosshairs, so it will be to your own detriment. Avoid brutal honesty, but try to be as sincere as possible.

So, as you approach a narcissist in an attempt to critique him/her, think long and hard about the structure of the conversation that is about to ensue. Have some sort of outline in your head before you start to speak. Preparation is the key, and you have to be able to anticipate and respond appropriately to some of the reactions that he/she may have. Walk through the conversation in your head try as much as possible to use positive language. You have to express yourself calmly and firmly because narcissists only respond to strength and not to weakness.

Come up with positive compliments with which to start your conversations. You can play into the narcissist's believes about himself or herself. If it's someone close to you, it's likely that you already know what it is that he/she wants to hear, so it wouldn't be too difficult to come up with compliments that they will respond to.

Your compliments can include a wide range of observations that you have made about the person lately, but you should try to give compliments that are closely related to the criticism that you want to dish out, because you don't want the criticisms to seem out of context (if the criticism comes out of left-field, the narcissist will know that your intention was always to be critical, and he/she will definitely hold it against you).

After you are done with your opening compliment, you want to use transitional words before you toss in your constructive criticism. Here, you want to make sure that your criticism sounds like a "by the way" without making it sound too insignificant.

Next, it's time to deliver the criticism. There is an art to doing this. You want the narcissist to feel like their way of doing things is almost perfect, but it would be completely perfect if they added this one minor correction. Since narcissists aspire to be perfect, they are likely to respond to your constructive criticism because they believe it would make them seem even more perfect in your eyes than they already are.

One technique you can use here is to make it seem as though the idea was his/hers all along. Since the narcissist wants to seem smarter than you, you can suggest several solutions to a problem (of those solutions, only one should be truly viable) and then leave it to him/her to make the decision as to which solution to implement for that particular situation. Narcissists love to take credit for other people's ideas, so you can structure the constructive criticism in a way that makes it easy for them to take credit for the idea of the change for which you are advocating.

You have to finish off by adding a few compliments so that you don't leave the narcissist with feelings of inadequacy. You can also try to paint a picture of how "awesome" things will be for the narcissist if he/she decided to incorporate your criticisms into his/her life.

There are a few things to remember as you use emphatic validation with a narcissist. First, you have to make sure that you pass your message across. It's a tight rope to walk, but it is doable. Secondly, you have to be careful about when and where you deliver your constructive criticism. It's okay to deal with some topics in the presence of other people, but there are topics that you must strictly bring up in private (the higher the potential for embarrassment, they more important it is for you to do it in private).

Chapter 5: Avoid Sharing TMI (Too Much Information)

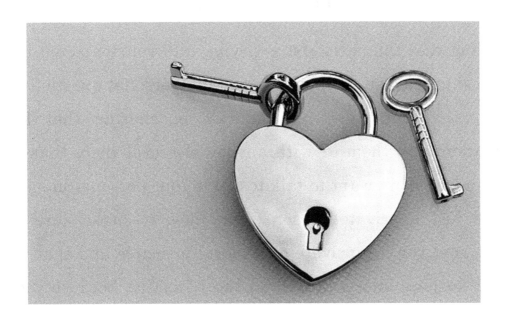

You probably already make a conscious effort to avoid revealing too much information when interacting with people at work, or even friends you don't fully trust. With narcissistic people, you have to filter your personal information even more than you are used to. Narcissists have the uncanny ability to use any kind of information against you, so don't trust them with any personal details.

You have to remember that the narcissist is going to actively seek out information about you under the guise of social discourse, but with bad intentions. They are going to pretend to be interested in you as a way to manipulate you and to elicit personal information from you. They'll do everything they can to put you at ease so that you let your guard down and spill all your secrets.

If you find that the narcissist is prying into your personal life, you have to shut it down. If they keep asking personal questions, make it clear that you have no intention of sharing that kind of information with them or with anyone else (tell them that it's not just them you don't want to talk to about your personal life and that you are just a private person). You have to make sure that it appears that you are private on general principle and that you are not just keeping information from the narcissist because you don't trust him/her.

Where private information is concerned, if you have identified someone as a narcissist, you have to tell all the friends and the family member that you confide in to keep your secrets from him or her. If a narcissist is out to get you and he/she finds that you are unwilling to provide personal information, he/she could decide to manipulate the people that are close to you in order to get it from them, so make sure that you swear your friends to secrecy where he/she is concerned.

Keeping your personal information from a narcissist is easier said than done. The fact is that these days, it's very easy to gain access to someone's personal information because we willingly share more than we need to online, and a narcissist who is interested in you can discern a lot about you from your social media accounts and the people in your social circles. So, you should be extremely careful about the kind of information that you divulge on social media platforms or even to the people around you. Even if there is no narcissist in your life right now, you never know when one might show up, and you want to avoid making it easy for someone to ruin your life.

To a narcissist, information is a weapon. Narcissists have perfected the art of turning even seemingly mundane facts into serious venom. They can make up lies or exaggerate your shortcomings, and even simple facts about your life can make them seem more credible when they are spinning their lies to mutual friends and acquaintances.

Let's say a narcissist knows which street or which building you live in. If he/she is malicious and out to get you, he/she could make up anything about you, and then drop in that simple fact. For example, a malicious colleague could say he saw you buying drugs on a corner of the street you live in. Because other people in your office know you live there, his made-up story will come across as significantly more credible than it would if he hadn't tossed in that information about you.

The point is that your threshold for what you consider as personal information should be a lot lower when you are dealing with narcissists than when you are dealing with other people. In fact, avoid sharing even the most obvious information with them if you can. If they are strangers, don't give them your phone number or tell them where you live out of politeness. If they are already in your life, try as much as possible to limit the new information that you give them.

If a narcissist finds out some personal information about you, there are things you can do to make that information less potent in case he/she decides to use it against you. If you discover that someone is a narcissist after you have already told them some details about yourself, try to think back and remember what it is they know about you, and then, in the spirit of transparency, make that information known to more people so that it has no potency if the narcissist decides to use it against you. At least this way, you can control how the information comes out.

Chapter 6: Don't Assume the Narcissist Cares About You

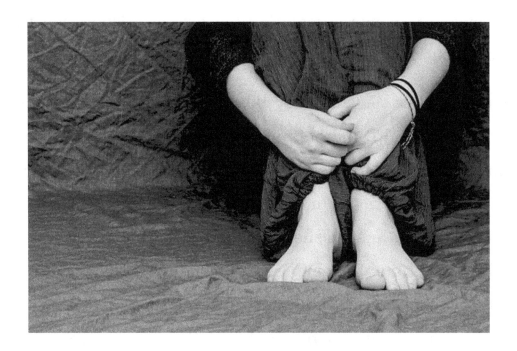

You can be forgiven for thinking that the narcissist cares about you because most humans have this innate desire to care about each other, and our default setting is to assume that others are also capable of caring about us. When you start out with the narcissist, he will give you the impression that he cares, but that is all an illusion because he wants something out of it. When the narcissist finally reveals his true colors, and you realize that he doesn't care, it can be a disconcerting experience, and you can even remain in denial about it for a very long time. That is because we are wired to look for the good in others, and when there is none to find, we keep digging deep. Don't waste your time that way — once you figure out that someone is a narcissist, it's time for the assumption that he cares to go out of the window.

If the narcissist is someone very close to you, he can start exhibiting cruel behavior that could be a major threat to you from a physical, emotional or even financial point of view. While you are still searching for the good in the person, he/she will keep taking advantage of you, and he/she will give you emotional wounds that could last a lifetime. In some cases, he/she could become physically violent. If you are a couple, he/she could also start spending all your money on things that benefit him/her without telling you, and then coming up with absurdly selfish explanations for this behavior.

Remember that the narcissist is quite devious, and he/she can take advantage of the fact that you think there is some good in him/her by feigning it once in a while to keep you on the hook. For example, if you are married to a narcissist who spends the cash in your joint accounts on things that benefit only him/her and put you in a financial quagmire, if he/she figures out that you are growing weary and you are about to leave, he/she may decide to spend some of that money on a "gift" for you, just to get you thinking again that maybe he/she isn't that bad.

An emotionally abusive narcissist may decide to buy you flowers once in a while just to get you thinking that maybe all is not lost in that relationship. You have to remember that these are just tricks that are meant to manipulate you so that you can stick around and suffer more abuse. In the narcissist's mind, he/she probably thinks that the occasional decent act negates all the horrible things that he/she does to you. Don't be fooled by the occasional kind acts.

You might ask, if a narcissist doesn't care, then why does he/she give me so much attention? This is a very confusing thing, and it has led many people to excuse the behavior of the narcissists in their lives for a long time. The truth is that for narcissists, attention is about control, having power over you, and manipulating you. Tricking you into thinking they care about you is like a sport to them, and they have a lot of fun with it. It's a sick game that they play with you to gain your trust. Once you trust them, they are going to manipulate you and bring out your insecurities so that you are somewhat dependent on them for emotional stability.

The sooner you accept the fact that the narcissist doesn't care, the sooner you will be able to get out from under his/her control, and the sooner you will be able to start healing and rebuilding your self-esteem. The longer you are stuck thinking the narcissist cares, the harder it will be for you to free yourself from his/her influence. There are people who have tolerated narcissists for so long, to the point that they have become numb to their own suffering and they have accepted the abuse as part of their existence. Don't let the narcissist break you, and don't lose perspective — you know a caring person when you see one, so don't make excuses for the narcissist.

Chapter 7: Don't Engage the Narcissist in Psychological Games

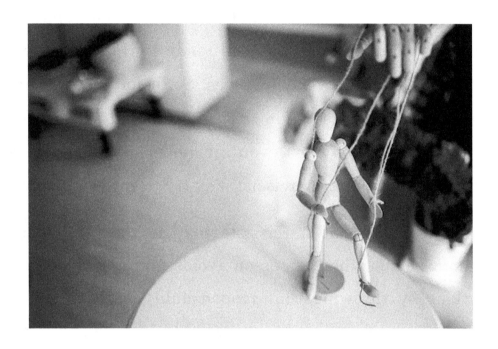

Narcissists are very good at initiating dramatic psychological games, often at your expense. They can stir up conflict between you and other people, and once you are at each other's throats, they'll pretend they had absolutely nothing to do with the situation at hand. So, if you sense that a narcissist is playing some sort of mind game with the intention of getting you to react in an aggressive way, you should take a step back.

Narcissists play games and start drama because they enjoy the chaos that ensues as a result of their machinations. When a narcissist starts a conflict between two people, he/she feels a sense of superiority over them — it feels like he/she is the puppet-master and you and others are tiny puppets ready to rip each other apart while he/she plays god over your lives. So, before you fall into the trap that the narcissist sets for you, and find yourself tangled in a drama whose origin you can't even remember, let's look at some of the common games that a narcissist may try to get you involved in.

One common game that narcissists play is the "emotional ping pong" game. This is where a person avoids taking responsibility for their actions by throwing that responsibility back to you. If the narcissist has done something reprehensible, instead of reflecting on his/her own actions and admitting wrongdoing, he/she will throw the ball back at you somehow. He/she could try to blame you, shame you, project fault onto you, or even outright deny doing something wrong, making you seem crazy for even pointing it out. If you care about him/her, you might find yourself believe the lie and even making excuses on his/her behalf.

Narcissists always love to play different variations of the 'game' where they make you seem crazy in front of other people. A narcissist could do something that indicates to you that they have malicious intent, but when you confront them, they can accuse you of having an overactive imagination, feigning innocence, or they can turn it around by accusing you of malice.

They could even get everyone around you to turn against you by making outrageous public accusations. Once you fall into that trap, you will start spinning out of control trying to prove to others that you are right, but that will only serve to prove the narcissist right. You have to learn to avoid reacting dramatically to the actions of a narcissist, and you have to be able to tell when you are being set up (with a narcissist, always assume that he/she is setting you up for something).

The most infuriating game that narcissists play is "gaslighting." This is where the narcissist flatly denies remembering something that you know perfectly well happened, and they insist that their memory is perfect and that you are the one who is mistaken. This is a very dangerous game, and it is surprisingly common in abusive relationships. If you stay for long with someone who "gaslights" you, in the end, you will start doubting your own perception of reality, and you will lose trust in your own recollection of events, your own reasoning, and intuition, and you will become a sitting duck for the abusive narcissist.

You have to remember to let the narcissist's games roll off your back because if you internalize everything that the narcissist tries to do to you if you fall into every trap he sets for you, if you give in and react in a dramatic way, in the end, you will lose.

If you play the narcissist's game for a long time, ultimately, you will suffer what pop-psychologists refer to as "death by a thousand cuts." This is where the narcissist will harm you in small ways over and over again until, in the end, he/she is able to destroy you completely. If you play the narcissist's games, he will destroy every part of you, by disparaging your accomplishments, destroying your ego and your confidence, casting doubt on your values and your belief system, and dampening your soul. If you let a narcissist have his/her way, he/she will turn everything that you are doing into a failure. If you are in a relationship, he/she will assign you the blame for everything that goes wrong, and take credit for everything that goes right.

Don't engage in the narcissist's drama. Don't play games. As a decent person, you will be inhibited by your rationality and your sense of decency. The narcissist won't play by any rules, so you can be absolutely certain that you will lose. The best way to win with a narcissist is to avoid playing his/her games altogether.

Chapter 8: Don't Second-Guess Your Decisions When Dealing With a Narcissist

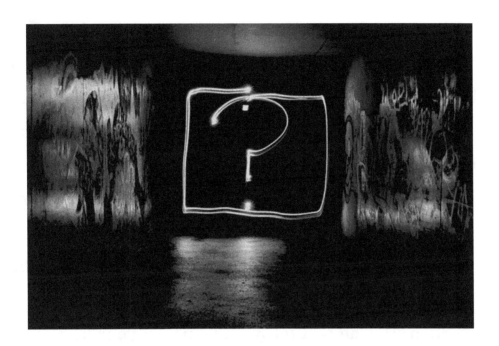

You don't need to justify yourself to the narcissist. When you interact with a narcissist, he/she will insist that you explain certain actions and choices that you have taken. You have to remember that your decisions are in your own best interests, and you don't owe the narcissist any explanation. Once you bother to explain yourself to the narcissist, it opens the door for him/her to then plant the seed of doubt on the decision that you have made with the intention of making you second guess yourself so that they can regain control over you. By all means, don't explain yourself. Let them know that you have already made a decision and that you are not seeking their input on the matter. It may seem rude, but it's necessary.

You can be certain that the narcissists will keep pushing for you to explain things to them. As we have mentioned in the last chapter, the only way to win a narcissist's game is to avoid playing it altogether. The narcissist will go out of his/her way to make you think that they are just trying to help, or that they are just making friendly conversation, but once you take the bait and offer an explanation for an action you have taken or a decision you have made, the narcissist will come up with a hundred different questions and observations, all of which are tailor-made to diminish your conviction. He/she will tell you it's not in your best interest to do what you are doing, you are not smart enough or strong enough to do it, or you need their help to see your plan through.

The narcissist knows that when you start doubting your perceptions and your convictions, you will have to rely on his/her guidance a lot more and that will give him/her control over you. When you get to the point where you don't trust your own judgment, then you will accept the narcissist's judgment, and he/she will be able to tell you what to do, and how to think and act at all times.

We have mentioned gas lighting in the previous chapter, but here, we will point out some of the signs that can indicate to you that you are being gaslighted, so that you are in a better position to stop doubting yourself and to avoid further manipulation.

First, the narcissist will start by telling a blatant lie. Since this is a person that you have known for a while and you trust to some level, the lie will throw you off balance, and you will start doubting things that are obvious. Next, the narcissist will deny things that they said, even if you can prove that they did. The more vehement their denial, the more you question your own reality!

The narcissist succeeds in gas lighting you because he/she wears you down over time. It's easy to think that you are too smart to get gaslighted, but the fact is that it doesn't happen instantaneously, it happens gradually, and one day you will wake up and find that you are so far gone. The way it works is that the narcissist will tell a small lie, stick with it and make you question your reality a little bit, but then you will decide that it's too small a lie to matter, so you will let it slide. The lies will then escalate both in magnitude and in frequency, and since you let the first one slide, you will have an easy time doing the same with the subsequent lies, until you get to the point where it's a norm. So, you shouldn't second guess yourself or let an obvious lie slide for even a second. Don't let the narcissist desensitize you to his/her lies.

Narcissists have perfected the art of turning things around to make it sound like you were the selfish one when it's clear that they are taking advantage of you. While you are still confused trying to decipher what it is that they are doing, they will make great strides towards altering your whole reality.

They will also send confusing signals by occasionally acknowledging some of your claims so that you begin to think that perhaps you were mistaken about the rest of the claims. For example, if you accuse the narcissist of 3 different things, he/she could cap to one and then deny the other 2, and this makes you think that he/she might be credible to some extent.

While gas lighting and other forms of manipulation can be infuriating and confusing, they are surprisingly easy to fall for, so you have to be vigilant. Your best bet is to stick to your guns and hold on to your reality. Don't let anyone talk you out of decisions that you have made, and by all means, don't ever substitute your perception for someone else's.

Chapter 9: Try Not to Take the Narcissist's Actions Personally

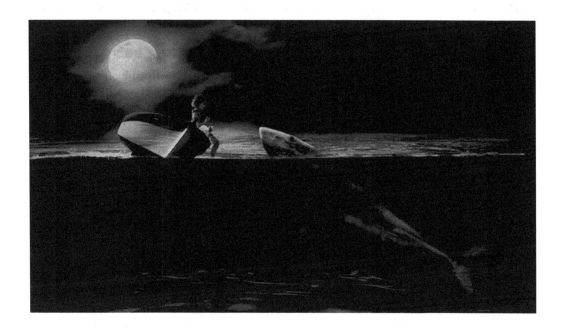

To the narcissist, it's never actually about you. To him or her, you are a pawn in a mind game that they are playing, and if you weren't there, they would be doing the exact same thing to someone else. Of course, this doesn't make their abuse less painful, but at least, it clarifies things for you. It means that your suffering isn't a result of any wrongdoing on your part.

When your relationship or your association with a narcissist finally goes south (as it is bound to do) you are going to start wondering how this person that you have known and trusted could have morphed into an entirely different and mean a person who you don't recognize at all. You will start thinking that maybe you did something to deserve their anger and their animosity. In your mind, you will feel that there has to be a rational explanation for what has happened. There is, of course, a psychological explanation for the things that are happening — but you can rest assured that you didn't play a part in making those things happen. They were just meant to happen, and they were never truly within your control.

The narcissist isn't hurting you or targeting you for a personal reason. You have nothing to do with it. The narcissist acts the way he/she does because that is the nature of the beast. It may seem callous, but it's true. The narcissist targeted you because you just happened to cross his/her path, or you just happened to be in their life.

If you have a narcissistic parent, you will realize that he/she treats both you and your siblings with the same level of narcissism (it may vary at different times, but everyone gets their share of abuse over the years). If you are in a relationship with a narcissist, you can be certain that he/she treated his/her former lovers the same way. In other words, the narcissist is an equal opportunity torturer.

This information doesn't make the suffering that you endured under the narcissist any less painful, but it has several important implications for you. First, it means that there is nothing wrong with you and that there is nothing that you did to deserve what the narcissist has done to you. Many people take the abuse of narcissists because they get accustomed to the suffering, and they start internalizing the idea that they might have done something to set off the abuse (most narcissists will try to blame you for lots of things, so if you let them, they can easily convince you that you have done something to deserve the suffering).

The second implication here is that there is absolutely nothing that you could have done to control the actions of the narcissists because those are his/her natural tendencies. Many people stay in abusive relationships with narcissists because they harbor the false belief that they can change them. Now that you know the narcissist's actions aren't personal, you understand that there is no way you can control those actions, so it's futile to believe that you can change a narcissist. That should clear your conscience and make it easy for you to end the relationship or the association with the narcissist (if you can).

The third implication is that the failure of your relationship with a narcissist isn't a commentary on your ability to give or receive love (the relationship was doomed to fail from the very beginning). So, as you leave, and as you move on, you shouldn't carry the baggage from that relationship onto the next one. The only thing you should bring along with you is your newfound ability to spot a narcissist from a mile away.

Don't delude yourself into thinking that the narcissist actually cares about you because what's happening is completely and utterly impersonal. We have mentioned that some narcissists are seducers, and they can make you feel like you are the center of the universe when they are looking to manipulate you. When this happens, it can be very tempting to ignore your instincts and everything you have learned so far about narcissists, but you have to stay strong and retain your rationality.

Chapter 10: Verify Any and All Claims That the Narcissist Makes

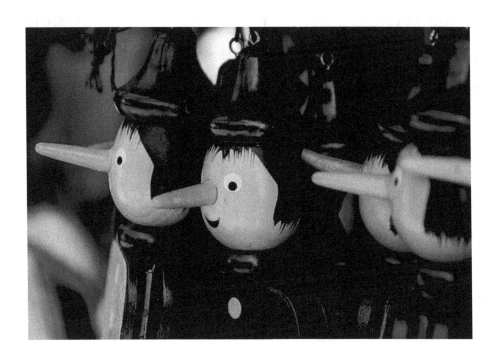

Narcissists are natural experts at lying. That is because they have learned to rationalize their lying, and they no longer feel any guilt the way ordinary people do when they mislead others. The next time the narcissist makes an outrageous claim, especially if it's about a mutual friend, take time to investigate the claim. Trust your own judgment about the person that the narcissist is making accusations against.

The most hardened narcissists could even pass polygraph tests while telling blatant lies because they are so adept at lying, that there is no cognitive dissonance that could cause a spike in their vitals. Some psychologists have come up with the hypothesis that narcissists lie about 80 to 90 percent of the time, and they even lie about petty and inconsequential things. Narcissists will only tell the truth when it benefits them.

To be safe, you have to treat every story you hear from the narcissist with a lot of skepticism. You have to start with the assumption that everything is a lie until you prove otherwise. As you do your realities check, here are some things that you need to pay attention to in order to figure out what the actual facts are and what the narcissist is lying about:

If the narcissist casts him/herself as some kind of hero in the story, you can rest assured that you are being lied to. We have already discussed how the narcissist has an overinflated ego, so as he/she creates a fictional story to manipulate you, he/she won't be able to resist the urge to be the hero in the story. If a narcissist tells you that a friend of yours was talking ill about you, he/she will claim to have been your only advocate in that conversation.

In an attempt to seem heroic and superior, the narcissist will also come up with stories about meeting (or being friends) with famous people, going to exotic places, or being an instrumental part of some groundbreaking accomplishment that you may be vaguely familiar with. These stories are often unprompted or out of topic, but the narcissist will bend over backward to make them seem relevant to the conversation that you are having.

As they try to manipulate you, one thing many narcissists tend to do is try to make themselves your best friend, so if the narcissist accuses a friend you have known for years of things that are clearly out of character, you should know that not only is he/she lying to you, it's likely that he/she is also telling similar lies about you to your friend in order to drive a wedge between the two of you.

In many cases, narcissists will also spin stories to cast themselves as victims even though they are the actual perpetrators. When a narcissist gets in trouble with a third party, he/she will come to you telling stories about being wronged, being treated unfairly, and how he/she went out of the way to be the bigger person. Even if you were there and you witnessed the whole thing, you will find the narcissist trying to convince you that things didn't go down as you thought and that you were the one who didn't pay enough attention.

If you catch a narcissist doing something wrong, he/she may also try to get out of the situation by spinning a story about how he/she was messed up as a child or in a past relationship and that his/her bad behavior is a consequence of past traumatic events. The narcissist may try to get you to empathize with him/her by saying how he/she has been working on this one weakness and how you shouldn't give up on him/her. This kind of lie often works in a relationship in which you already feel invested. That kind of "confession" can make anyone seem endearing.

If a narcissist tells you that he is coming from a dark place, he is sorry, and he is on a journey to change his life, you should be greatly alarmed. If you let the narcissist off the hook because of a story like that, he is going to use the same story over and over again, and the more times you let it go, the harder it would be for you to take a different stance in the future.

When narcissists spin a story, they are going to inject a few half-truths into that story to make it seem more credible to you. You should be keen to note if the narcissist adds "facts" into the story, including places you are familiar with, days you vaguely recall, or people you used to know. The intention is to make you more inclined to believe him/her. You should pay attention to the unnecessary details that the narcissist throws into the story, and the detail he/she brings to your attention with a bit of emphasis, then if you can, fact-check those details. More often than not, they are all lies.

Chapter 11: Don't Compete With the Narcissist

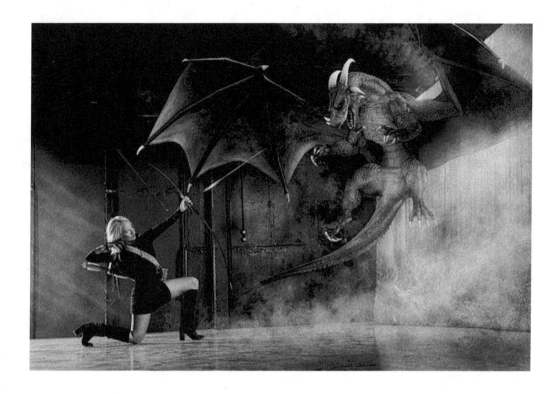

You don't want to put yourself on the spot when you are dealing with a narcissist, so the worst possible thing that you can do is try to compete with him/her on trivial things that don't actually matter to you. Narcissists take trivial competitions seriously, and if you try to one-up them in any way, you will end up losing.

There is one simple reason why you are going to lose. The narcissist is ready and willing to cross lines that you as a reasonable person will never dream of crossing. You don't operate under the same rules of decency, so if you try to one-up a narcissist, your own conscience will keep you from winning.

Another important thing to note is that even if you one-up a narcissist and you win by all objective standards, the narcissist will just declare himself the winner anyway and there is absolutely nothing you can do about it. Victory against a narcissist will never be as sweet as you hoped because he will never acknowledge it or give you any respect as a result of your victory. He will just tell people the opposite thing happened, and you will then seem petty if you try to insist that you were victorious.

When dealing with a narcissist, your first instinct should be self-preservation and trying to one-up the narcissist won't help you with that. If you try to compete with a narcissist, you are only going to make yourself more of a target, and that could lead to your destruction. We are not suggesting that you be submissive and let the narcissist walk all over you, we are saying that you should be above it, and you should avoid getting down and dirty with the narcissist. Narcissists want to feel like they are winning over you, but if you don't try to one-up them, you are essentially telling them that you don't care about their silly games, and this may make them go out and try to find someone else over whom to assert their dominance.

If you avoid one-upping a narcissist, he could stop bothering you because it's just not fun for him. For example, if a narcissistic colleague starts telling you how smart and knowledgeable he is, you can just say "good for you" and carry on with your work. Because he wants to feel in control, the fact that you seem calm and unfettered will tell him that he may be out of his depth here, and he could proceed to find someone else to bug in order to feel superior. However, if you respond to his assertions by telling him where you went to school and how much experience you have, he will take that as a challenge, and he will never seize trying to prove he is smarter than you.

Once you try to one-up a narcissist, you are in a game that is going to last for the remainder of your relationship or your association with the narcissist. The only way that game is going to end is if you admit defeat, so the best thing for you is to never get into it in the first place.

When we one-up people in normal social situations, it's because we want them to think highly of us, but the thing with narcissists is that no matter how accomplished we are, they are never going to think highly of us or to give us the respect we deserve. So, if you really think about it, there is no upside to one-upping a narcissist. Only misery can come out of the decision to do such a thing.

It's possible to one-up a narcissist unintentionally, without ever realizing it, and when this happens, the consequences can be disastrous. There are things that you can do avoid inadvertently one-upping a narcissist. For example, when you are talking to other people about things that you have accomplished recently, you can avoid using the word "I" and instead use the word "we" so that the narcissist doesn't feel slighted. If the narcissist is a colleague with whom you have worked on a project, when you report to your boss in his presence, don't say "I solved the issue," instead, say "we solved the issue." The narcissist likes to hog credit, but he would rather share it with you than not get it at all.

Chapter 12: Get Away From the Narcissist

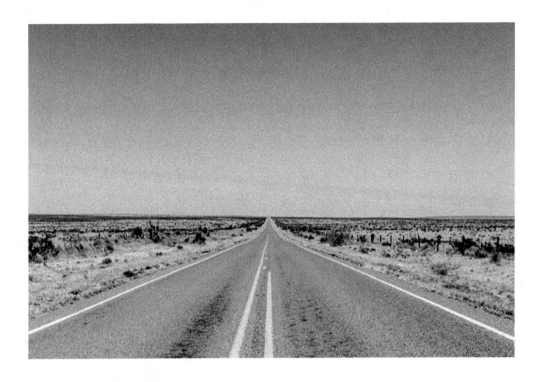

You have to get away from the narcissist because staying is not good for you in the long-run. However, there are situations where the narcissist in question is a vital part of your life, and it's utterly impractical for you to leave him/her completely. For instance, he/she could be a spouse with whom you have kids, a family member, or a colleague in your department. In such cases, you can try to put as much distance between the two of you as possible while at the same time trying to limit the harm that befalls your kids, your other family members or your career respectively.

If your lives aren't already intertwined, you can break up with them, leave them, and avoid contacting them altogether. Remember that they didn't really care about you, so don't worry too much about how they are going to feel after you break up.

Don't bother explaining too much detail about why you are leaving. Remember that if you take the time to justify yourself, they are going to try to talk you out of it. Break up in a public place and leave, never to return. Don't agree to be friends with them or to hang out in the future, no matter how insistent they are.

Some psychologists even suggest that you should break up with narcissists over the phone because there is no way of telling how in-person meetings are going to go. When you avoid contact with the narcissist, tell him that he is not welcome into your home, and block his number from your phone. If you leave the tiniest window open, he is going to find a way to crawl back into your life. Don't do any lingering goodbye. Just say your piece and leave.

There are always going to be some mutual friends who are going to vouch for the narcissist and tell you that you made a mistake leaving him. These friends may mean well, but they certainly don't fully understand how much you have been suffering under the thumb of the narcissist. With them, you have to make it clear that the narcissist is persona non grata, and the cost of bringing him up during your conversations is that they will lose your friendship. Tell them that you don't want any updates on the narcissist's life, and if they still talk to him, they shouldn't tell him anything about you either.

When you leave a narcissist, that very same day, write down exactly why you left him. In your journal, put down the rationale for your decision, and all the reasons why being with him was a bad thing for you. The purpose of this is that when the narcissist comes crawling back into your life and tries to manipulate you, you can refer back to your journal and remember why it's vital that you stay away from him. We have talked about gas lighting and how a manipulative narcissist can get you to question your own sanity, so having contemporaneous records of your thoughts and feelings can help you stay grounded on the truth.

If you successfully get away from a narcissist, hopefully, he/she will move on quickly, find someone else torment, and leave you alone. Because the narcissist never really cared about you in the first place, he won't be too hung up on your relationship, so don't question your decision when you see that he/she has moved on too quickly and you start to worry that you may end up alone. Being alone is better than being with someone who sucks the life out of you.

Chapter 13: Ignore the Narcissist

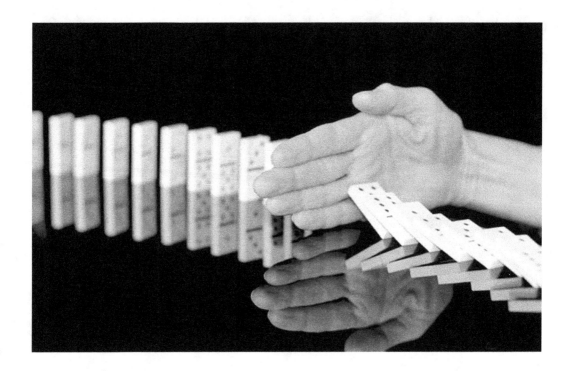

The narcissist lives to trigger emotional reactions in people because, in their minds, that gives them some sense of power. If a narcissist causes you to lose control over your emotions, it gives him a lot of satisfaction. When a narcissist attacks you verbally, ignoring him can drive him crazy.

You have to understand that narcissists crave attention, so ignoring them hurts them more than anything else. They want to be acknowledged and validated; that is why they start with the conflict in the first place. When a narcissist targets you and destroys your life, your natural instinct will be to get back at him/her by reacting angrily and emotionally, but if you do that, you are only playing into his/her hand.

It may not seem so at first, but over time, you will realize that ignoring the narcissist is actually much more satisfying than engaging with him/her because then, even to third-party observers, the narcissist will just seem like a petty person who likes to pick fights with people, and you will seem like the mature adult who is able to rise above it all.

The narcissist wants to control you and to assert dominance over you, but you have to remember that people can't take power from you. You actually have to give it to them. A narcissist can only have dominance over you if you relinquish control to him/her. As we have mentioned, you are guaranteed to lose if you play the narcissist's game, and that is when he/she is actually capable of dominating you. By ignoring the narcissist, you blatantly refuse to play his/her game, and then he/she has no means with which to get close enough to have any form of control over your life.

In as much as ignoring the narcissist hurts him/her; remember that you are doing it for yourself and for your own peace of mind. When you choose to ignore a narcissist, don't be preoccupied with the effect that the lack of attention has on him/her. Focus on doing something worthwhile for yourself. If after ignoring the narcissist, you are still obsessed with how he/she is reacting to it, then you are still under his/her control, and you are relinquishing your power to him/her.

When you ignore an ex who is a narcissist, don't turn around and start stalking him on social media to see if he is miserable. Now that you have regained control, you should focus on detoxifying from the narcissist's influence and training yourself to be more vigilant in the future.

If the narcissist is someone who is in your life permanently, ignoring him/her is going to be a regular thing, so you have to train yourself so as to get better at it. Ignoring a narcissist is more than just avoiding responding to their taunts. It's about learning to stop caring about their opinions and their criticisms. The first step is to restrain yourself from responding to them even if their comments hurt you, but after that, you have to work on yourself to get to the point where what they say rolls off you like water.

Remember that although you have no control over what the narcissist says, you have control over how much importance you associate with the things he/she says or does. Once you figure out that a person is a narcissist, you should make a conscious effort to stop attaching any actual meaning or value to their words and actions. Just regard them as malicious, and assume all their actions towards you are ill-conceived. That way, you are less likely to get hurt by them.

When you ignore a narcissist, you have to keep your safety in mind. Some narcissists tend to turn aggressive or violent when you deny them attention, so you have to be careful not to be anywhere with them without witnesses present. Ignoring a narcissist makes him/her feel that you have slipped away from his/her control, and in a desperate effort to regain that control, you never know how they are going to lash out. You have to be a lot more cautious and a lot smarter going forward because the narcissist is going to bring his/her "A" game in order to regain control over you. Keep ignoring them, and no matter how hard they come at you, don't relent, not even slightly.

Chapter 14: 10 Things a Narcissist Will Always Do In a Relationship

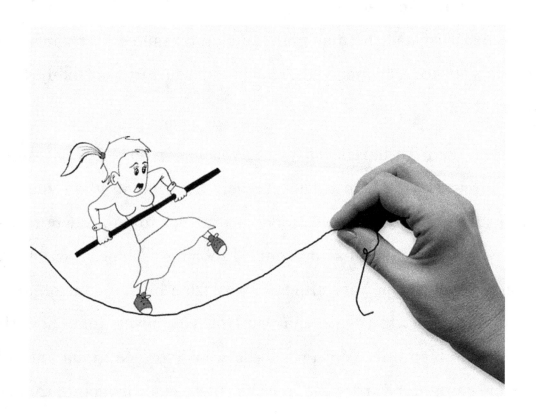

You can be able to tell if the person you are in a relationship with is a narcissist based on the kind of behavior he/she exhibits throughout the duration of your relationship. Ideally, you want to be able to figure out if your boyfriend, girlfriend, or even an acquaintance has narcissistic tendencies as soon as possible so that you can sever ties with him/her before you are too invested in that relationship. Here are ten things that a narcissist will always do in a relationship.

He Will Try to Charm You

As we've mentioned throughout the book, narcissists can be quite charismatic and charming when they want something from you. If you are in a relationship with one, he will go out of his way to make you feel special in the beginning so that you trust him enough to let your guard down. As long as you are serving the purpose he wants you to serve; the narcissist will give you a lot of attention and make you feel like you are the center of his world. If someone puts you on a pedestal during the early stages of your relationship, you should pay more attention to the way they act, just to see if they are faking it.

He Will Make You Feel Worthless

After you have been hanging out with a narcissist for a while, you will notice that when you have any sort of disagreement or argument, his first instinct is to dismiss you in a way that makes you feel worthless. He will criticize you in the sort of contemptuous tone that will make you feel dehumanized. When you disagree with ordinary people, you always get the feeling that your opinion matters to them, but with a narcissist, that is not the case. All the things about you that the narcissist claimed to like when he was charming you will somehow turn into negative attributes, and the narcissist will portray himself as a "saint" for putting up with those attributes.

He Will Hog Your Conversations

Narcissists are in love with the way people perceive them, so they will take every chance to talk about themselves. Whenever you try to have a conversation, the topic is always going to change, and it will suddenly be about them. It's never a 2-way conversation with a narcissist unless he is trying to manipulate you into thinking he cares about you. You will get to a point where you really struggle to get him to hear your views or to get him to acknowledge your feelings. When you start telling a story about something that happened to you at work, you will never get to the end of it because he is going to start his own story before you are done with yours. If you make comments on certain topics of conversation, your comments will be ignored, dismissed, or even corrected unnecessarily.

He Will Violate Your Boundaries

From very early in the relationship, the narcissist will start showing disregard for your personal boundaries. You will notice that he violates your personal space, and he has no qualms about asking you to do him favors that he has by no means earned. He will borrow your personal items or even money and fail to return it, and when you ask, he is going to say that he didn't know it was such a big deal to you — the point is to make you seem petty for insisting on boundaries that most decent people would consider reasonable.

He Will Break the Rules

The narcissist will break the rules that you set for your relationship, and other social rules, without any compunction. The problem is that sometimes, we are initially attracted to rule breakers because they seem to be "bad boys" or "rebels," but those traits are in fact tale-tell signs of narcissism. A person who breaks social norms is definitely going to break relationship rules because relationships are essentially social contracts. If someone is trying to charm you, but in your first few interactions, you observe that he cuts lines, tips poorly, disregards traffic rules, etc., you can be certain that you are dealing with a narcissist.

He Will Try to Change You

When you are in a relationship with someone, they are definitely going to change you in a few minor ways (often unintentionally). However, when you are dealing with a narcissist, he is going to make a deliberate and perceptible effort to change you, and more often than not, it won't be for the better. He will try to break you, and he will try to make you more subservient to him.

You will find yourself making concession after concession, until, in the end; any objective observer can tell you that you are under his thumb. He will cause you to lose your sense of identity so that you end up being a mere extension of him. When you get out of that relationship, you will find it difficult to figure out who you are as an individual because he would have spent the entire duration of the relationship defining and redefining you.

He Will Exhibit a Sense of Entitlement

The narcissist will demonstrate a sense of entitlement for the most part of your relationship. At first, he may seem generous and considerate just to draw you in, but after that, you will see his entitlement rear its ugly head. He will be expecting preferential treatment all the time, and he will expect you to make him a priority in your life (even ahead of your own career or your family). There will be a clear disconnect between what he offers and what he expects, and he is going to want to be the center of your universe.

He Will Try to Isolate You

Any narcissist who wants to control you and make you subservient to him understands that you have a support system of friends and family who won't stand by and let him harm you. So, one of the things he will do once he has faked affection and earned some of your trust is he is going to try and isolate you. He will insist that every time you hang out, you shouldn't bring anyone along. He will make up lies to drive a wedge between you and your friends. He will play into the conflicts that exist between you and your family members to make you lean on them a lot less. If you let him get rid of your support system, he will have free reign, and you won't stand a chance against his manipulation.

He Will Express a Lot of Negative Emotions

Narcissists trade on negative emotions because they want to be the center of attention. When you are in a relationship with one, he is going to be upset when you don't do what he wants, when you are slightly critical of him, or when you don't give him the attention he is looking for. He is going to use anger, insincere sadness, and other negative emotions to make you insecure, to get your attention, or to gain a sense of control over you. If someone you are dating throws a tantrum over minor disagreements or when you aren't able to give him attention, it means that he has a fragile ego, which is a clear sign that he could be a narcissist.

He Will Play the Blame Game

This is perhaps the most common indicator that you are in a relationship with a narcissist. He will never admit to any wrongdoing, and he will always find a way of turning everything into your fault. When anything doesn't go according to plan, he will always point out your part in it, even if he too could have done something to change the outcome of the event. He will never take responsibility for anything, and when he takes action to solve a mutual problem that you have, he will always make it clear that you owe him.

Conclusion

Thank you for making it through to the end of *Dealing with a Narcissist*, let's hope it was informative and able to provide you with all of the tools you need to retake control of your life from the narcissist that has been ruining it.

The next step is to start implementing the lessons that you have learned here in a smart and strategic way so that you can loosen the narcissist's stranglehold on your life without making yourself more of a target.

In this book, you have discovered how the mind of a narcissist works, and what makes him/her tick. When you start dealing with the narcissist in your life, you have to take these lessons to heart. You have also learned how you can identify different types of narcissists, so make sure that you figure out what kind of narcissist you are dealing with, so you can come up with the best strategy for dealing with him/her.

You have also learned how to create boundaries and stick to them when dealing with narcissists, and how to use emphatic validation when you want to criticize a narcissist. Make sure that you don't overlook this advice because it could make your life a bit easier.

You should also remember the "don'ts" that we have discussed in detail within the book. Make sure that you don't share too much information with the narcissist; you don't assume that the narcissist cares about you, you don't play the narcissist's games, you don't second guess yourself when dealing with a narcissist, and you don't assume that the narcissist's actions are personal.

There is a big difference between reading about how to deal with a person or a problem, and actually doing it in real life. When you are dealing with an actual narcissist in real life, you are going to feel scared and under pressure, and it's easy to forget the right approach when it comes to handling the situation. When you confront the narcissist, take a deep breath, and remember that you stand your best chance of getting your way when you are calm and collected.